MW00356081

PENGUIN BOOKS

Use It Or Lose It

The legendary Peter Snell, born in Opunake in 1938, is one
of the greatest athletes of all time. He won three Olympic
gold medals at 800 and 1500 metres in sensational fashion
in the 1960s, displaying a powerful finishing burst that has
perhaps never been matched by anyone. He has held eight
world records and was voted New Zealand's sportsman of
the twentieth century. Snell left New Zealand in his early
30s to study in the US and is now an associate professor
at the Department of Internal Medicine at the University
of Texas Southwestern Medical Center and director of
the UT Southwestern Human Performance Center. He
lives in Dallas with his wife Miki.

Garth Gilmour was born in Dunedin in 1925, and
from 1941 until 1986 worked as a journalist on various
newspapers throughout the country and in advertising
and public relations. He began writing books in the
1960s and *Use It Or Lose It* is his nineteenth. His first
book was with Arthur Lydiard, the leading coach and
inventor of jogging. Under his influence Garth gave up
smoking and took up jogging. He has run five marathons
and is an occasional golfer and recreational cyclist. He
lives in Auckland with his wife Kay.

Use It
Or Lose It

Be Fit, Live Well

Dr Peter Snell PhD and Garth Gilmour

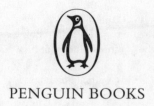

PENGUIN BOOKS

PENGUIN BOOKS

Published by the Penguin Group

Penguin Group (NZ), cnr Airborne and Rosedale Roads, Albany,
Auckland 1310, New Zealand (a division of Pearson New Zealand Ltd)
Penguin Group (USA) Inc., 375 Hudson Street, New York, New York 10014, USA
Penguin Group (Canada), 90 Eglinton Avenue East, Suite 700, Toronto,
Ontario, M4P 2Y3, Canada (a division of Pearson Penguin Canada Inc.)
Penguin Books Ltd, 80 Strand, London, WC2R 0RL, England
Penguin Ireland, 25 St Stephen's Green, Dublin 2, Ireland
(a division of Penguin Books Ltd)
Penguin Group (Australia), 250 Camberwell Road, Camberwell, Victoria
3124, Australia (a division of Pearson Australia Group Pty Ltd)
Penguin Books India Pvt Ltd, 11, Community Centre, Panchsheel Park,
New Delhi – 110 017, India
Penguin Books (South Africa) (Pty) Ltd, 24 Sturdee Avenue, Rosebank, Johannesburg
2196, South Africa

Penguin Books Ltd, Registered Offices: 80 Strand, London, WC2R 0RL, England

First published by Penguin Group (NZ), 2006
1 3 5 7 9 10 8 6 4 2

Copyright © Peter Snell and Garth Gilmour, 2006
Copyright © illustrations remains with the individual copyright holders.
The publisher has made every reasonable effort to locate the copyright holders of the
images in this book. If you have any information regarding the copyright of images
in this book please contact the publisher.

The right of Peter Snell and Garth Gilmour to be identified as the authors of this
work in terms of section 96 of the Copyright Act 1994 is hereby asserted.

Designed by Mary Egan
Typeset by Egan Reid Ltd
Printed in Australia by McPherson's Printing Group

All rights reserved. Without limiting the rights under copyright reserved above,
no part of this publication may be reproduced, stored in or introduced into a
retrieval system, or transmitted, in any form or by any means (electronic, mechanical,
photocopying, recording or otherwise), without the prior written permission of both
the copyright owner and the above publisher of this book.

ISBN 0 14 302060 9
A catalogue record for this book is available
from the National Library of New Zealand.

www.penguin.co.nz

Contents

Introduction

THINK OF the Third Age. What mental picture do you form from those two words? Depending on your age as you read this, it will vary dramatically. Some, probably the younger among you, will imagine old people sitting in rows, occasionally dribbling a bit; others may see white heads, grey heads, dyed heads and bald heads on top of sagging bodies. Still others may picture busloads of goggling tourists seeing as much as they can of the world before they die, or streams of people with lined but intent faces heading purposefully back into the world's higher education institutions.

The permutations are endless. And a grim thought is that a lot of people are never going to fit any of those images because they are not going to make it.

Let's try to be rational about this Third Age thing. The First Age covers childhood, the teens and maybe the early 20s – those carefree and often careless years. The Second Age is dramatically different: it's the age of career paths, marriage, mortgages, children, home and security building – a small mountain of responsibilities for most.

The Third Age probably comes as a smudge on the horizon of your sea of life as you enter your 50s. Consciously or subconsciously, you begin to gear yourself towards the inevitability of retirement and a new way of living without the rigours, rewards and disciplines of your years of employment. Your children have grown and gone, you have achieved all or as much as you could of your ambitions. In short, if the First Age is all about receiving and the Second is all about giving, the Third is all about self-fulfilment. Now is the time to do the things you always wanted to do. It is often also the time when you have your first awareness of your mortality, when it enters your consciousness that you are more than halfway to wherever you are going next. It adds urgency to that need to do those things you always wanted to do. So, how? What now?

It's your choice

When that smudge on your horizon becomes a ship and sails into your port, will it be a rust-streaked tramp steamer or a luxury liner glowing with lights and laughter? It can be your choice.

So far, all through your life, you have been faced with a seemingly endless series of choices to make. Think about it. You get up in the morning, having first made the choice between getting up and lying in a little longer – and it begins. What to wear? What to have for breakfast? Whether to even have breakfast? Will it rain or won't it? Do I take the car or chase the bus? Have I time for the bus?

On it goes, all day and into the night when you make the penultimate choice: when do I go to bed? Now because I'm tired or later because I want to watch that TV show? The ultimate choice, of course, is made in bed and depends totally on your personal circumstances.

This choosing between options has been going on since you were born into this crazy world, since you first decided to accept, or reject, the food your doting mother was thrusting at your clenched-mouth face, be it breast or bottle. This preferential food selection process follows us through life, every day of our lives.

Our interaction with other people is largely based on or governed by choices we make. Do we like or hate the kids next door? Auntie Mame? The grocer who offers us lollies with an unctuous smile? The younger sibling, born when you were two, who threatened your centre-stage role in the family?

And, in most cases, we determine how long we live, how happily we live – or how soon we die – from the options we choose. Now, as the mysterious Third – and probably last – Age looms, what we choose to do about it may be among the most vital decisions we have ever been asked to make.

It is an alarming fact that our life expectancy, which has been increasing for centuries, is now in danger of beginning to regress, purely because far too many of us have been making far too many wrong decisions.

The good and the bad

Those are the decisions this book is mainly concerned with: to explain the consequences of the everyday decisions we make about our health, whether they vary from better to worse; to outline how the best decisions should, and can always, be made; to set out the methods by which the wrong decisions you may already have made can be countered; and to show you that making the right decisions, even against your preferences, can be an enjoyable process as well as achieving long-term benefits.

Modern medicines and medical, physical and nutritional sciences have gone a long way towards giving us the basis for living longer and more healthy lives. But it is typical of our penchant for wrong choices that we have found incredible ways to foil all that good work. We build bigger and faster cars, which can make bigger messes when they or, more likely, their drivers fail. We smoke and drink to excess. We have perfected the art of polluting our environment. We indulge in interminable violence, warfare and allied mindless mayhem in the name of religions, lost causes and tribal or racial differences. We have, as a consequence of our changing, loosening lifestyles, been confronted with the scourge of Aids. We have developed a range of designer drugs that deliver to the user every experience from temporary euphoria to brain damage and death. We are the victims of booming criminality, which ranges from petty theft to the cruel suppression, exploitation and starvation of nations of helpless men, women and children.

These examples do tend to be aberrations. The norm is for people to live out their lives, maybe moved but mainly untouched by major catastrophes and demonstrations of inhumanity: they grow up, find jobs, get married, have children, look placidly forward to the future when the children have left the nest and impending retirement will be a pleasant prospect.

Turning the key

But right there, in the security, maturity and practicality of that enviable normality, lie the keys to whether we finally make that goal of retirement and, if we do, whether we can actually enjoy it. How we use those keys to protect, enhance – and perhaps extend – our final years is entirely over to personal choice. And commitment.

It has been predicted that within the next quarter of a century or so four times as many people as today will become centenarians. Reaching the very ripe old age of 120 is now considered not impossible; nor is it totally inconceivable that one day people can look forward to living for 200 years – assuming that, by that time, there is still somewhere to live and some reason to live there. These are interesting thoughts and theories which, perhaps, should not be dismissed out of hand, even if they are unlikely to materialise in our lifetimes.

To some extent, it is daydream stuff and it tends to obscure the hard, fact-founded reality that, far from living longer lives, a great proportion of us will live needlessly shorter ones.

The fat boom

In the US more than half the population is significantly overweight. They are fat, if not classifiably obese. In New Zealand government-funded health research has declared that more than half the nation's children now exceed their recommended bodyweight.

These are incredible developments given the boom in interest in personal fitness, well-being and wellness that has occurred in the past two or three decades. Overweightedness is becoming an alarming issue all round the world, even among countries which have had a long tradition of leanness.

Westernisation has a lot to do with it, bringing to the rest of the world the doctrine of easy living, fast and convenience foods, and the television-watching slump – the constantly munching and drinking couch potato bombarded with exhortations to eat and drink more of, mostly, the wrong kinds of food. Machines are continually being developed that take the labour out of labour. Far more people work sitting down; far fewer use the muscles that their parents and grandparents did. They're even working on a gadget to cook fast food faster, as if we no longer have time to relax over a meal. It is ironic that the very things designed to free us from drudgery and give us more time for relaxation and pleasure are actually condemning us to earlier function loss or death because we have become too careless about looking after ourselves or our families.

Man or mouse potato?

The dependence on the computer has given rise to a new phenomenon – the mouse potato, young or old, who spends hours of his or her week sitting or, more often, slumped in front of the screen while the great free, fresh outdoors goes to waste.

There is an irony in the enthusiasm with which the US (and many other nations) has seized on concepts of physical fitness and well-being, while at the same time leading the world in the promotion of the very antithesis of those two desirable objectives. And the other pioneers of the age of electronic ease, the Japanese, are experiencing a similar problem of decreasing physical effort and increasing poundage.

In 2005 New Zealand TV watchers were presented with a news item showing a fatties' contest, involving bellyflops in a swimming pool, somewhere in the US. Contestants had to weigh more than 110kg and the one who made the biggest splash won a prize. The contestants were fat and obese people, rather than muscled Tarzans, but the reward wasn't a weight-loss programme; it was $1000 and 1000 cream-filled doughnuts.

While gross fatness is being glorified and rewarded, the way ahead to better, longer living seems to be a road paved with landmines but it is still a road worth following. It can be easy and enjoyable. All you have to do is step around the landmines and move briskly onwards.

We are the same as you

Peter Snell is the product of his choices. As a teenager he could have been an outstanding tennis player. Or a great golfer. He chose to be a runner and, at 21 years of age, became the most dramatic and greatest middle-distance athlete the world has yet seen. He has three Olympic gold medals (two at 800 metres, one at 1500 metres) and ran eight world records to prove it. His king-hit for his opponents was a finishing surge so violent that he threw chunks of the track back in their faces and put metres on them in a few strides.

At the end of his running career, he could have returned to his futureless work as a cigarette company PR and sports foundation director, the job that had enabled him to concentrate on his running, or found some other employment back in New Zealand. But, despite his own recognition that he had been an unspectacular, even dismal, scholar, he elected to pursue an academic life to find out about, and enhance, those physical and physiological elements that make human performance tick.

With the same single-mindedness that marked his running, he spent the next few years, starting from behind scratch, qualifying himself as an authority on the subject and becoming a major contributor to the understanding and advance of athletic prowess. He succeeded with a brilliance that paralleled his running. He had spent 1971 studying at Loughborough University of Technology's Department of Ergonomics in England but, in 1974, he became a full-time student at the University of California in Davis, graduating in 1977 with a BSc in human performance. Four more years at Washington State University gained him a PhD in exercise physiology.

He is now associate professor in the Department of Internal Medicine (Cardiology Division) at the University of Texas Southwestern Medical Center and director of the UT Southwestern Human Performance

Center in Dallas, where he moved in 1981 after four years as research and teaching assistant at Washington State University.

He is an inaugural inductee of the International Scholar-Athlete Hall of Fame at the University of Rhode Island, is New Zealand's Sportsman of the twentieth century, is patron of the New Zealand Parkinson's Society, is a past president of the Dallas Division of the American Heart Association, was on the US Olympic Committee Sports Medicine Council from 1990 to 1995, was a 1990 member of the USOC Nutrition Advisory Committee and is a member of the American College of Sports Medicine and of the US Track and Field Scientific Advisory Committee.

New age, new interest

His earlier work at Dallas centred on elite athletic performance and cardiovascular and muscle adaptation to training. He then made the decision that his next career aim should be to do something about making the inevitability of ageing a transition in life that should not be feared, should not be depressing, but which should be a doorway into a new kind of enjoyment, fulfilment and wellness. His specialty now is exercise, cardiovascular disease and ageing.

He says he became interested in ageing because he is now old himself – if you regard the mid-60s as old. He wants to be an advocate for people over 50. It's a great age and he has been thoroughly hacked off by people who say that old people don't have much to offer. Older people created the society in which young people now live and, he believes, are entitled to some respect for their achievements and their continuing ability to contribute wisdom to the world.

'I don't feel washed out and ineffective because I am now in my 60s,' Snell says. 'I'm just getting smart enough to know what's going on and I'm comfortable with who I am. A lot of young people are not and are desperately struggling to make their marks and define themselves.

'Old people are relaxed. I think we know who we are, which gives me the belief that I can make a difference in educating people to do more exercise, take better care of themselves and, as an outcome, live fuller, healthier, happier Third Age lives.'

Not Superman

Peter Snell is not a superman. He is an ordinary man. Sure, he has specific qualities, mental and physical, which he has employed to make himself as great and successful as he can be. But that could be said of most people. The difference, perhaps, is the level and intensity of application. Now in his 60s, Peter Snell is a Third Ager, still demonstrating the legacy of his earlier fitness, strength and mental determination, but also concerned that he, like everyone else approaching, entering or already in that tertiary stage of life, should enjoy it to the full as long as possible.

The 0.02 second choice

I have been a Third Ager for a long time. Although now in my 80s, I have made more choices than I care to remember because many of them were wrong ones. But one decision, the fastest I ever made, stands out as the pivotal point of my life. Soon after international coaching guru Arthur Lydiard returned from the 1960 Rome Olympic Games with his three medal winners, Snell (800 metres gold), Murray Halberg (5000 metres gold) and Barry Magee (marathon bronze), I, as a sports reporter for the *Auckland Star*, interviewed him. In the course of our conversation, Lydiard said he had received many offers from publishers to write a book on his revolutionary training methods. But, he said, he couldn't write a book.

'Get someone to help you,' I suggested. 'Would you be interested?' Lydiard asked. My answer to that question took an estimated 0.02 seconds, possibly a world record at the time, and my life changed for ever.

I moved from an 80-a-day cigarette smoker to a jogger and eventual marathon runner and have been co-author with Lydiard ever since, producing more than a dozen variations of our original book, *Run to the Top*, including two specifically on jogging for international markets. I also co-authored the biographies of Snell and Halberg and other world-famous athletes, have just completed a book on the transformation of the Lydiard running system into a highly successful system for swimming-training, and was able to complete a biography of the amazing Lydiard just before his death, at 87, in Houston, Texas, on 12 December 2004.

I keep fit on the saddle of a bicycle and in other activities so that I can continue working and enjoying golf, swimming and the good life of the Third Age.

The flip side

There have been hiccups. I have knackered knees from my late and overenthusiastic running burst, a suspect spine from a vertebral fusion following a squash accident in 1972, a colon shortened by the removal of a sizeable cancerous tumour in 1985. But I believe I also have a life substantially lengthened by my association with Lydiard and his runners so I owe it to them not to waste it or spoil it. One of my aims is to play a round of golf to my age. Just once will be enough. I may have to live to be 90, or even 100, but that doesn't matter. Having the target is what is important. It's a reason to stay fit, keep swinging.

There's also a 176km bike race round Lake Taupo, in the heart of the North Island, that lurks in a corner of my mind as something I would like to master. I tried in 2003 but, undertrained to a serious degree, I capitulated after 100km of more than 12 testing hills and growing headwinds. It was only the second time since 1949 that I had pedalled a bike for that distance. But maybe one year I'll go back to Taupo. Perhaps next year. Possibly never. Again, I believe it is almost as important to keep it in mind as an incentive as it is to actually get the opportunity to do it.

Now, after 40-plus years, I have reunited with Peter Snell to produce this book as my contribution to what I have always believed the ageing world desperately needs – simple, sensible and thorough guidance in the art of growing old gracefully, usefully and without an excess of effort.

I, too, am an ordinary person who happened to make at least one choice that was absolutely right for the rest of my life.

Peter Snell and I want everyone to make the choice that is absolutely right for the rest of *their* lives.

Reading this book may well teach you more about your own body but everything you learn is important in understanding how your personal assemblage of blood and bones and bits works and how it can be maintained or improved.

A final word: this book is aimed at achieving a happy Third Age but it is not just for Third Agers. How you enjoy that third stage and for how long is something you must consider right through life. Whatever your age, start now.

Garth Gilmour

CHAPTER ONE

Getting Started

WILLIAM SHAKESPEARE, in *As You Like It*, mused on the life cycle of using it and losing it with a whimsical wisdom that is a warning to us all that our lives are finite and fraught.

> All the world's a stage,
> And all the men and women merely players.
> They have their exits and their entrances,
> And one man in his time plays many parts,
> His acts being seven ages. At first, the infant,
> Mewling and puking in the nurse's arms.
> Then the whining schoolboy, with his satchel
> And shining morning face, creeping like snail
> Unwillingly to school. And then the lover,
> Sighing like furnace, with a woeful ballad
> Made to his mistress' eyebrow. Then a soldier,
> Full of strange oaths and bearded like the pard,
> Jealous in honour, sudden and quick in quarrel,
> Seeking the bubble reputation
> Even in the cannon's mouth. And then the justice,
> In fair round belly with good capon lin'd,

With eyes severe and beard of formal cut,
Full of wise saws and modern instances;
And so he plays his part. The sixth age shifts
Into the lean and slipper'd pantaloon,
With spectacles on nose and pouch on side;
His youthful hose, well sav'd, a world too wide
For his shrunk shank, and his big manly voice,
Turning again toward childish treble, pipes
And whistles in his sound. Last scene of all,
That ends this strange eventful history,
Is second childishness and mere oblivion,
Sans teeth, sans eyes, sans taste, sans everything.

Growing old is a function most of us manage to perform but how we do it varies wildly and widely. We are, with advancing years, the targets of numerous and varying aches, pains, diseases and ailments as our bodies remorselessly decide to degenerate. We can't stop the process in its tracks but we can do much to slow down, even reverse, some of ageing's symptoms and causes, and we can do it as simply or as demandingly as we choose. The main ingredients – and perhaps the only ones you need – are determination, willpower and patience.

Approach with caution

Peter has always liked the method of having goals that are realistically achievable and then moving on to a new, more difficult goal – defining mini-goals that are steps towards a larger goal. With this technique, success is more frequent and has a positive effect on motivation. When Arthur Lydiard told Peter, as a 19-year-old, that his track performances would improve with increased endurance, he set a mini-goal to make the Auckland cross-country team and worked diligently throughout the winter without any thought of the following track season or anything beyond that.

In spite of understanding how this process works for physical activities, Peter felt he was less successful in applying the techniques as a writer. For example, in writing the material for this book, he could find excuses not to write and weeks would pass without any progress. James Michener said that, even though he may not have felt inspired, he sat down at his typewriter every day. Maybe in physical activities there is less need to be inspired but, as the Nike ads insist, 'Just do it'.

In the realm of fitness, let us say that you would like to be able to do 50 push-ups off the toes. Seems impossible; right now you can only do five before the arms start to quiver and refuse to do another. No problem. Muscles recover fairly quickly and after doing those five push-ups, move on to 20 bent-knee sit-ups, come back with another five push-ups and then repeat a third time. Later in the day, maybe at the office, do another series of two sets of five and then repeat again a couple of times in the evening. This is an easy way to accomplish 50 push-ups in a day. Next day, try to do six or seven at each session, but maintain the daily volume at 50. You will be amazed at how your triceps (the muscle group on the back of the upper arm) will respond to this regular challenge.

In a similar manner, a goal of jogging 8km may be quite formidable to a novice, yet, using the same principles as above, this distance can be achieved easily. Start by walking initially and then intersperse short periods of slow jogging with one- to two-minute walks in between. In a relatively short time you will be able to increase the jogging phase and eventually cut out the walks. Avoid the temptation to jog or run faster before you are able to jog the full distance without having to walk. This was the approach of Lydiard athletes new to distance running – first achieve the distance at a comfortable pace, then improve speed, rather than trying to run fast initially and increase the distance.

Apart from the appropriate clothing and footwear, all you need are those three ingredients of determination, willpower and patience. Simple as that.

Simple tips

Here are some ideas on how you can apply yourself without great effort:

- Do something on your goal *every* day.

- Try something new if current methods aren't working.
- Repeat methods that *do* work.
- Listen to successful people's advice.
- Keep your mind open.
- Picture your goal constantly.
- Expect the best.
- Commit yourself to your goal.
- Every day rewrite your 'things to do today' list after reviewing your goals.

Many people find excuses for not achieving goals. The most common, especially for failing exercise goals, is 'I don't have enough time'. Translated, this means 'I am not organised enough' or 'It is not important enough to me and therefore motivation is low'. Peter is currently conducting an exercise study on HIV-positive patients aged 40 to 50 to determine if exercise can reduce the negative side-effects of Aids-preventing drugs on fat metabolism and insulin resistance. Without exception, they are highly motivated to do the programme, which has the potential to make them look and feel better. Older people, 60-plus, with medical problems such as diabetes, often seem more fatalistic towards their situation and more readily give up.

Keeping in mind the need for patience in whatever you have decided to do to hold ageing at bay, consider these questions:

- Could you spend more time on your goal, work more effectively at it? Check that you are really doing your best.
- Have you been given advice you haven't heeded but which, on reflection, might help?
- Are you trying reasonable approaches, as suggested earlier?

The battle against ageing is a mental one, too. There is little point in keeping the body fit and well if you don't also exercise your brain. This is another aspect this book will explore more closely later.

Let's add another ingredient to the central trio, determination, willpower and patience. Whatever you decide to do to stay physically and mentally as fit as you can, make it fun. Not work. *Fun.* Just as people tend to work better at jobs they enjoy doing, so your anti-ageing activities should be tailored to give you enjoyable rewards.

You'll improve physically and you'll improve psychologically. The world will seem brighter.

What is ageing anyway?

We'll come back to these issues in more detail later but, meanwhile, what exactly is ageing? The simple but facile answer is, of course, growing old. But scientists, physiologists, philosophers and sometimes-fanciful theorists spend vast amounts of time and energy in going a great deal deeper than that. It is a fascinating subject with considerable attention paid to cellular theories and research, which have shown that the human body's cells have a programmed number of divisions or doublings that they go through before beginning the process of dying (apoptosis). Cells cultured from older individuals go through fewer doublings than those taken from a newborn so, clearly, there are mechanisms of ageing at the cellular level, the details of which are yet to be fully determined.

Several theories, involving topics such as cross-link, free radical, immunology, genetic ageing and telomeres – a word which many of the best dictionaries don't yet explain – have been advanced as a result of prolonged and intensive studies, but none of them is particularly helpful at this stage. That's one of the troubles with theories – they take an age to verify and, more often than not, are not useful. Like so much research, solutions are always just around the corner.

The cross-linking hypothesis is based on the observation that with age, our proteins, DNA, and other structural molecules develop unnecessary attachments or cross-links to one another. These links or bonds, formed through a process called glycosylation, decrease the mobility or elasticity of tissues. Diabetics with chronically high glucose levels are at greater risk for glycosylation, which leads to cataracts, stiff arteries and other problems.

Free radicals, which may be caused by radiation, environmental pollutants, chemicals, sunlight, stress, and smoking, are reactive molecules that damage tissues, including our DNA. Damage to our vital genetic material causes mutations that can lead to cancer and other diseases.

Telomeres, for instance, are necessary for life and function as they prevent our chromosomes from unravelling. However, after some 80 cell divisions, the telomeres become so short that the cells stop dividing, enter a state of senescence – a nice way to say they grow old – and die. Human cells produce telomerase, an enzyme that repairs damaged telomeres, but this stops early in life and so creates a time bomb that kills most of us in our 70s and 80s.

Researchers into telomeres are trying to find a way of preventing this time bomb going off. Some of their work looks promising, but has had unfortunately exaggerated effects. For instance, in 1998, UT Southwestern Medical Center scientists in Dallas (Peter's racquetball buddies Woody Wright and Jerry Shay) discovered that telomerase has an astonishing ability to immortalise certain kinds of cells which, normally, die quite quickly. The announcement of this discovery led the press to produce the inevitable, overcharged spin that ageing was about to become an artefact of the past, even though the scientists never claimed that telomerase had anything to do with human lifespan. The discovery became a sensational story because it appealed to our ancient and eternal interest in cheating death and living for ever.

A huge, lucrative industry caters to that interest, offering pills, potions and powders meant to reverse the effects of ageing. These fixes do not, will not and cannot work, say scientists. They reject the claims of 'prolongevists' who believe the fountain of eternal youth is about to play for us.

Short of medical interventions that manufacture survival time, there is very little any of us can do to extend the latent potential for longevity that was present at conception. In the aggregate, some scientists say, we have already passed the far limits of our life expectancy, evidenced by the fact that many of the diseases that plague us, such as certain cancers and neuromuscular disorders, are the expression of genes that have long been with us but were not often manifested because we did not live long enough for them to become a problem. Now, of course, we do. And they do.

Adding still more years will not necessarily do anything to improve quality of life. The better approach is to guard our health during the years that are ours and to regard all claims to immortality and life extension, no matter how attractive, with a sceptical eye.

Despite the astounding increase in longevity made during the 20th century (in the US, the mean age went from 45 at the beginning of the century to 78 by its end), it is doubtful that we will witness any dramatic increase in the foreseeable future. In fact, the leaping obesity problem throughout the world suggests the opposite. Our lifestyle is making it more difficult for us to reach happy old age comfortably but it is making dying sooner a whole lot easier. Another rational argument is that it would be far more difficult to increase life expectancy by curing illnesses in elderly persons than it has been to nudge that expectancy upwards by reducing infant mortality.

Any increase above 85 would require biomedical breakthroughs in our ability to affect the basic processes of ageing itself and not just in our ability to treat diseases. This pessimistic evaluation, while controversial, injected a much-needed shot of realism into a field in which some researchers were seriously predicting life expectancy would soon rise above 100. Maybe it will, one day, but let's not get carried away yet.

The quest for the causes of and 'cures' for ageing will go on and so will the efforts (both legitimate scientific research and bogus claims for alternative therapies) to prolong life and delay ageing. It has been established that natural selection promotes health during the reproductive period but contributes little benefit over the age of 60. It is only in the past 100 years that most humans have begun to outlive their reproductive years and many of the diseases of ageing are a recent development.

Medical intervention can 'manufacture' extra time but that is as far as it goes. Healthy life, rather than simply longer life, should be the goal. It is achievable. It is not wishful thinking.

Our genetic heritage has left us with bodies rather like the cars that are designed to perform flawlessly in the Indy 500 – if their drivers insisted on continuing many miles beyond the end of the race their parts would inevitably begin to fail.

Ageing itself is not a disease that can be cured. Genetic manipulation and antioxidants may affect the ageing process but some scientists decry the often outrageous claims now made for antioxidants. They counter ancient myths of longevity, and diets and dietary supplements aimed at averting ageing with the strong argument that proponents of such treatments, in fact, have themselves died at the expected age and of the usual causes.

University of Chicago scientists researched three types of pro-longevity myths: antediluvian legends that people once lived very long lives; Hyperborean myths that, in particular places, people live very long lives; and 'fountain' legends of substances that allow people to live very long lives. These legends persist, they say, in today's promises of life expectancies of 120 years or more.

So, the battle for better living goes on. The search for some kind of Holy Grail continues. But waiting for someone to find it won't help you now.

Only you can do that.

CHAPTER TWO

Fat Facts

FOR THE FIRST TIME in 1000 years, future generations are likely to die at a younger age than their parents, a US *Journal of Medicine* study reported in March 2005. It predicted that life expectancy, which has been rising for centuries, will drop by as much as five years in the next few decades.

The reason: increasing numbers of obese and overweight adults will bring the figure down as they die early from conditions such as diabetes, heart disease and cancers.

The obesity problem is bad right now but will get worse when today's obese and overweight children hit middle age. It will also worsen because the Eastern world is now following the Western world's obesity pattern, largely due to the adoption of the Western fast-food and couch-potato cultures in the wake of growing prosperity in places such as Japan, Korea and China.

The US study cited above, which also found that factors such as pollution, pandemic influenza and the use of tobacco could also hit life expectancy, has been criticised by other researchers as 'excessively gloomy'. A United Nations study, for example, suggests life expectancy could reach 100 in many countries by 2300.

But the latest statistics show that about half a million adult New

Zealanders are obese – twice as many as 25 years ago – while an estimated one in 10 school-age children is overweight and half of those are obese. Studies have estimated that obesity can reduce a person's life by five to 20 years.

A 2003 Life in New Zealand survey found 43% of men and 27% of women to be overweight; while 10% of men and 13% of women qualified as obese.

The facts and figures show us the sad state of the world's health today. So does this picture of our evolution:

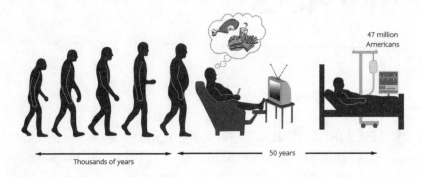

Figure courtesy of Dr Roger Unger, UT Southwestern Medical Center.

Overweight or obese?

Many people have a natural tendency to get fatter as they get older. But the tendency is getting out of control and shows no signs of abating. Since 1960 the number of overweight and obese Americans has continued to increase. Now about 55% of adult Americans – some 98 million people – are categorised as either overweight or obese. Another scary fat figure in America is that at least 40 million people – about one-quarter of all adults and one in every five children – are obese. Crowd scenes on television lend credence to this unwelcome statistic: bulging bellies and backsides on the move.

Every year obesity is estimated to cause at least 300,000 unnecessary deaths in the US at a cost to the country of more than $US100 billion. It is associated with high blood pressure, adult-onset diabetes, high fat (triglyceride) levels in the blood, and has become the second leading cause of death. Fat stored in adipose tissue (storage site for fat) is okay. but when it invades other tissues, such as muscle and the heart, the most vital muscle of all, the function of these tissues is impaired.

The following facts show the spread of obesity around the world. In the US obesity rates have reached epidemic proportions, including among children. Excess fat is a problem in the rest of the world as well.

The US

- 58 million overweight; 40 million obese; 3 million morbidly obese.
- Eight out of 10 over 25-year-olds are overweight.
- 300,000 premature obesity-related deaths a year (400,000 tobacco-related).
- 78% of Americans are not meeting basic activity level recommendations.
- 25% lead completely sedentary lives.
- There has been a 76% increase in type 2 diabetes in adults 30 to 40 years old since 1990.
- 80% of type 2 diabetes is related to obesity.
- 70% of cardiovascular disease is related to obesity.
- 42% of breast and colon cancers is diagnosed among obese individuals.
- 30% of gall-bladder surgery is related to obesity.
- 26% of obese people have high blood pressure.
- 4% of children were overweight in 1982; 16% were overweight in 1994.
- 25% of all white children were overweight in 2001.
- 33% of African-American and Hispanic children were overweight in 2001.
- Hospital costs associated with childhood obesity increased from $35 million in 1979 to $127 million in 1999.
- One in four overweight children is already showing early signs of type 2 diabetes (impaired glucose intolerance).
- 60% of children already have one risk factor for heart disease.

- Between 8% and 45% of newly diagnosed cases of childhood diabetes are type 2, associated with obesity.
- 4% of childhood diabetes cases were type 2 in 1990; now the rate is approximately 20%.
- Of children diagnosed with type 2 diabetes, 85% are obese.
- Americans eat 300 to 400% more fat than they should.
- Each day the average American eats the equivalent of one whole stick (113g) of butter.
- Nearly 50 cents of every dollar spent on food is spent on eating outside the home. With super-sized portions, dining out is the perfect recipe for fast weight gain.
- An estimated 70% of Americans take insufficient exercise.

Scotland
- One in five children aged 12 is clinically obese.

Australia
- 47% of women and 63% of men are overweight or obese. If this trend continues, by 2010 around 70% will be above their healthy weight range.

New Zealand
- More than half the adult population is overweight (35%) or obese (20%).
- If current trends continue, 29% of all adults are likely to be obese in 2011.
- One-third of children aged between five and 14 are overweight (21%) or obese (10%).
- 27% of Maori men and 28% of Maori women were obese in 2003.
- 26% of Pacific Island men and 47% of Pacific Island women are obese.
- 1000 obesity-related deaths occur each year (double the annual road toll).

Europe

- Obesity is common, especially among women and in southern and eastern countries.
- Obesity prevalence ranges from 10 to 20% for men and 10 to 25% for women, following a 10 to 40% increase in the last decade.
- In the UK obesity has more than doubled since 1980.

Africa

- Little data are available. The emphasis has been on undernutrition and food security rather than overweight and obesity but regional studies indicate both are rising. In South Africa 44% of black women in the Cape Peninsula were found to be obese.

Middle East

- There are limited data but indications are of a high prevalence of obesity. Obesity among women is higher than in most Western countries.

The Caribbean

- Obesity is a significant problem; 49% of black women have been identified as overweight.

South America

- A survey in Brazil, the only one conducted in Latin America in the last decade, indicates obesity is prevalent, especially among lower-income groups. The dietary deficit problem is changing to one of dietary excess.

Japan

- Obesity among men has doubled since 1982. Among women aged 20 to 29 it has increased 1.8 times since 1967.

China

- Obesity is increasing, and is more common in urban areas and among women.

Pacific nations

- Obesity, long regarded as a symbol of high social status and prosperity in Polynesian and Micronesian societies, has increased dramatically in the last 20 years.
- In 1991, 75% of urban males in Western Samoa were obese. In 1986, 23% of schoolchildren in Tonga were obese.

References: Wellness International Network Ltd; Nutrition Australia (2000); 1997 New Zealand National Nutrition Survey; 2002/3 New Zealand Health Survey.

It is particularly disappointing to see the rise of obesity in teenagers all over the globe. The number of fat cells in the body is determined by how fat you are during development. Thus, obese children develop more fat cells, which makes it more difficult for them to control weight later in life. Adult-onset obesity occurs as a result of fat cells increasing in size rather than number.

Nations once seen as naturally lean are now showing similar evidence of galloping overweightedness. Japan is a classic example and is concerned about what is happening to its national waistline. The reality of spreading girths and doubling chins doesn't make them acceptable.

An intriguing side-effect of the weight-growth problem is that airlines are being forced to shed seats, spend more on fuel and fly more slowly, according to a report in October 2001 from the US Federal Aviation Administration. US Air Force doctor Major Donato Borrillo has estimated that the average North American passenger now weighs 85kg, which he calls 'a sign of obesity of epidemic proportions'. If the passenger weight guideline rises by 3kg, a jumbo jet with 400 passengers will be officially carrying 1.2 tonnes too much.

In New Zealand, in 1995, passengers usually weighed between 72.5kg and 77kg but that average is now believed to have reached 80kg or more. This means that airlines, especially those using small planes, are having to be more careful about safe take-off weights. Passenger capacity was reduced by one or two seats more than two years ago.

Air New Zealand in 1998 issued figures showing its cabin crew averaged 82kg and technical crew 94kg – not because they were bigger but because they were fatter.

In November 2004 Southwest Airlines in the US angered the country's 'fat acceptance' lobby by asking larger passengers to buy a second seat. The crash of a commuter plane that killed 21 people in North Carolina was blamed on the passengers' larger-than-average weight. Other figures released in 2005 found that the average American's weight gain of 4.5kg during the 1990s cost airlines an extra 1325 million litres of fuel, worth some $400 million. With unconscious irony, the report said airlines' financial bottom lines were being hurt – by Americans' bigger bottoms.

Before you dash to the bathroom scales, you can calculate your personal body mass index (BMI) because this is used as one definition of the state you are in weightwise. You calculate your BMI by dividing your bodyweight in kilograms by your height in metres squared or consult the table on the following page.

The National Institutes of Health and National Heart Lung and Blood Institute's Clinical Guidelines on Overweight and Obesity (June 1998) consider overweight to be reached when BMI is between 25 and 29.9. Over 30 and you are obese. But several factors can distort the findings. Very muscular people and pregnant or lactating women, for example, can produce misleading BMI results and, in our opinion, there should be two scales – one for sedentary people whose muscles are atrophied and one for active people (especially in the case of those middle-aged and older as ageing reduces total blood volume and muscle and bone mass).

Two people can have the same BMI, but a different body-fat percentage. A bodybuilder with a large muscle mass and a low body-fat percentage may have the same BMI as an obese person (BMI >30) because BMI is calculated using weight and height only and ignores differences in muscularity.

BMI is widely used by physicians and in large-scale studies of obesity prevalence. It is at best a crude estimate of fatness. The accuracy of the following table would be enhanced by asking a simple question about regular physical activity, to adjust for exercise-induced muscularity.

Determining your body mass index (BMI)

BMI (kg/m²)	19	20	21	22	23	24	25	26	27	28	29	30	35	40
Height (cm)	Weight (kg)													
147	41	43	46	48	50	52	54	56	59	61	63	65	67	69
150	43	45	47	49	52	54	56	58	61	63	65	67	70	72
152	44	46	49	51	53	56	58	60	63	65	67	70	72	74
155	46	48	50	53	55	58	60	62	65	67	70	72	74	77
157	47	50	52	55	57	60	62	64	67	69	72	74	77	79
160	49	51	54	56	59	61	64	67	69	72	74	77	79	82
163	50	53	55	58	61	63	66	69	71	74	77	79	82	85
165	52	55	57	60	63	65	68	71	74	76	79	82	84	87
168	53	56	59	62	65	67	70	73	76	79	81	84	87	90
170	55	58	61	64	67	70	72	75	78	81	84	87	90	93
173	57	60	63	66	69	72	75	78	81	84	87	89	92	95
175	58	61	65	68	71	74	77	80	83	86	89	92	95	98
178	60	63	66	70	73	76	79	82	85	89	92	95	98	101
180	62	65	68	72	75	78	81	85	88	91	94	98	101	104
183	64	67	70	74	77	80	84	87	90	94	97	100	104	107
185	65	69	72	76	79	83	86	89	93	96	100	103	107	110
188	67	71	74	78	81	85	88	92	95	99	102	106	110	113
191	69	73	76	80	83	87	91	94	98	102	105	109	112	116
193	71	75	78	82	86	89	93	97	101	104	108	112	116	119

The men in the table below have the same height, weight and BMI, which at 30.5 is classified as 'obese', but their body-fat percentage is greatly different.

BMI compared to body-fat percentages

Height	Weight	BMI	% Fat
180cm	101kg	30.5	8
180cm	101kg	30.5	35

Our suggested additional column to the right would put the body builder from the previous paragraph in the 'overweight' rather than 'obese' category and Peter Snell (BMI 26.5, 16% fat) would move from 'overweight' to 'normal'.

Or better still there should be two BMI ranges for sedentary people and very active people. See the table below:

BMI and physical activity

BMI standard	Weight status	BMI for active people
Below 18.5	Underweight	Below 20.5
18.5–24.9	Normal	20.5–26.9
25.0–29.9	Overweight	27.0–31.9
30.0 and above	Obese	32 and above

Recommended body-fat percentage

The following recommendations are based on population studies derived from published measurements of over 50,000 people.

		Ages				
		20–29	30–39	40–49	50–59	60+
Male	% Fat	7–17	12–21	14–23	16–24	17–25
Female	% Fat	16–24	17–25	19–28	22–31	22–33

This table allows for the reality that as people get older they get fatter. Theoretically, there is no reason why body-fat percentage should increase with age other than through a reduction in activity levels.

At the 1964 Olympic Games, Peter was 77.1kg and 179.1cm for a BMI of 24.1 – almost overweight. Today's measurements, 83.9kg and 177.8cm, place him at 26.5. In other words, he is defined as overweight and would become obese at 94.3kg.

As one of those fortunates who never change weight significantly, Garth Gilmour's BMI is 23.6. He weighs 68kg and stands 169.5cm tall.

Body weight in kilograms according to height and body mass index

The best definition of obesity is 25% fat for men and 30% fat for women. The ideal for men and women ranges from 13 to 15% and 23 to 25% respectively, with no adjustment for age. The 'gold' standard for estimating body-fat percentage is using total body density derived from the technique of underwater weighing (which yields body volume from which the density and then body-fat percentage is calculated). A less accurate but useful technique is to measure skin and subcutaneous fat folds at certain parts of the body (thigh, abdomen, hip, etc.) using callipers (can you pinch an inch?). Devices that measure the electrical resistance of the body are showing up in health clubs, but the results can vary widely depending on where the measurements are made (between hands, legs or, preferably, one hand and the leg on the opposite side) and the state of hydration (resistance is lower in water-containing tissues, such as muscle, and higher in fatty tissues). For instance, the fat percentage of a person carrying excess upper-body weight will be overestimated if the resistance between left and right hands is used.

Not all the underlying causes of obesity are known yet. It is accepted that overweight and obese people don't necessarily eat more than thin people but are more likely to be less active so their net energy intake exceeds their net energy output. Reduce the intake, increase the expenditure and you're on your way out of the fat-race.

A low basal metabolic rate (BMR) can be a cause of obesity. That rate is the amount of energy needed to maintain vital body functions at rest (heartbeat, breathing, etc.) and it partly determines energy requirements. Peter often has people requesting this measurement in his lab in the hope that their obesity may be due to a low BMR, but only rarely does this turn out to be the case. Heredity factors can have some bearing; the children of obese parents are 10 times more likely to be obese compared with the children of parents of normal weight. Some hormonal disorders such as excess cortisol production (Cushing's syndrome) or hypothyroidism are accompanied by obesity but these are uncommon.

The hormone leptin is made by a specific gene found in fat cells. Leptin influences the appetite centres of the brain and reduces the urge to eat. It also seems to control how the body manages its store of body fat. Since leptin is produced by fat, leptin levels tend to be higher in obese people than in people of normal weight, but it is likely that obese people aren't as sensitive to the effects of leptin and may be overproducing the hormone in an unsuccessful attempt to compensate. Research is focusing on why leptin messages aren't getting through to the brain in obese people.

Various studies have shown that leptin levels drop after low-kilojoule diets. Reduced leptin increases the appetite and slows the metabolism. This may help to explain why crash dieters usually regain their lost weight once they revert to normal diets.

The pituitary gland in the brain produces growth hormone, which influences an individual's height and contributes to bone- and muscle-building. Growth hormone also affects metabolism. Researchers have found that growth hormone levels in obese people are lower than those in people of normal weight and that exercise enhances growth hormone production.

The menopause and the contraceptive pill have been blamed for obesity in women but the reality here is that the weight gain is small and is mostly due to water retention.

Stress, on the other hand, one of the counselling profession's boom industries, can cause people to eat more and pile on the kilos. So can anger and sorrow. As an interesting corollary, physical inactivity tends to accompany all three of these emotional responses.

Cut it out

You can treat obesity and overweight in several ways: the surgical options of liposuction, stomach stapling and the wiring of jaws; stringent slimming diets; exercise; and what the experts call behavioural modification, which simply means changing your way of life and being strictly in control of how you change to replace the negatives with positives.

The surgical possibilities are drastic. The diets – if you can determine which is the right one – call for strong willpower combined with possible distaste for what you may be reduced to eating. But exercise is easily attainable and need not be strenuous to be useful.

A general principle of dieting is to take in less energy than the energy you expend, forcing your body to take the energy deficit from that stored excess fat. The target would be to shed about 1kg a week, so it could be a long programme, even if it is strictly followed. Diets that get that fat off much faster tend to be short-lived.

Exercise can begin with the simplest proposition: a walk to the local dairy instead of riding in the car, or taking a regular walk around the block, along the beach or through the park. But it will need a purposeful and steady growth of energy output to achieve any rewards. A wide range of options for achievable solutions will be spelt out in finer detail later.

Modifying the way you live is a challenge, particularly if you are overweight or obese because of some emotional problem. You need to record all the food and drink you consume, when and with whom, and events and moods that trigger the need to eat, until a pattern of activities and negative emotions can be identified and a method developed to block the overeating habits.

Out of the Hale Project, headed by KTB Knoops, in September 2004 came the suggestion that the secret to a long life could be as simple as a Mediterranean-style diet, which may not be good tidings for Atkins-style foodies. The 10-year study, which followed 2339 people aged 70 to 80 from 11 European countries, was one of the first to look at the individual and combined effects of diet and lifestyle in older people and found a 23% reduction in overall deaths during a decade among those who adhered to a Mediterranean diet.

Similar reductions were found among those who consumed moderate amounts of alcohol, primarily wine (22%), engaged in regular physical activities (37%) and did not smoke (35%). Putting all four together – diet, alcohol, exercise and not smoking – effected a 65% reduction in overall deaths. Considering that all four are achievable and not unpleasant, the reported result is noteworthy.

The study, published in the *Journal of the American Medical Association*, also found that walking 3km a day significantly reduced the risk of dementia in older men.

Diana Kerwin, an assistant professor of medicine at the Medical College of Wisconsin, said the study showed that at age 70 you can still add some lifestyle habits that affect longevity.

The lead author of the Mediterranean diet study, KTB Knoops, a researcher with the division of human nutrition at Wageningen

University in the Netherlands, said the reductions came from lower rates of death from heart disease, cancer and other causes.

In the Atkins diet, for example, red meat typically is not restricted but carbohydrates are cut dramatically, including those from potatoes, many fruits, grains and alcohol. It focuses on weight loss whereas the Mediterranean diet aims to maintain a stable weight.

Should any doubt remain that the world is becoming conscious of its expanding girth and decreasing life expectancy, the US Department of Agriculture wiped it away when it launched, in May 2005, its new food pyramid and website. In its first 24 hours, MyPyramid.gov took 48 million hits and temporarily crashed.

The new pyramid is a formula designed to be customised according to age, sex and activity level and the critics of the old pyramid heaped praise on the new ploy on the block.

But, once the hype died down, some nutritionists found a few bugs in the system. One pointed out that if you wanted to translate your customised diet into meals you would have to take your measuring cups and calculator to the restaurant with you. The new pyramid offers a deluge of information, recommending portion sizes down to fractions of an ounce – but it doesn't take into account such vital information as an individual's height and weight. Harvard University food guru Walter Willett said, 'It has gone from being so simple it doesn't say anything to being so complicated that it's not useful.'

Another problem: the personalised pyramid is available only online, which means it excludes many low-income people, who are the very ones with the least access to good food and have the most problems associated with its lack. The USDA said it planned to reach the underprivileged populations with a non-Internet version.

Yet another: the emphasis on dairy-based foods is heavy but many minorities are lactose intolerant, and a large body of nutritionists, including Willett, don't see dairy as a necessary part of a complete breakfast – or any meal at all, for that matter.

So, in the way that desperate people will grasp at any straw – even one blowing in the wind – MyPyramid will be in fashion until it is discredited or some better easy-fix idea comes along. It's still better to strive for a balance between sensible eating and adequate exercise, for which you need no measuring cups or calculators – just plain common sense, commitment and willpower.

Meanwhile, a Stanford University study has thrown a curveball at MyPyramid with a finding that coloured vegetables, which include red capsicums, carrots, broccoli and red cabbage, are a dietary winner. This study found that a low-fat diet rich in vegetables, fruits, whole grains and beans has twice the cholesterol-lowering power of conventional low-fat diets, which often contain the wrong nutrients. This resulted from a focus on the negatives – what to avoid, rather than what to include.

Stanford's study team tested 120 adults between the ages of 30 and 65, all with moderately high low-density lipoprotein (LDL, the 'bad' cholesterol) with levels of 130 to 190. The desirable level is 100. Sixty-one of the volunteers ate a conventional low-fat diet, which included frozen waffles, turkey sausage sandwiches and frozen pizza. The other 59 ate a plant-based diet, including wholegrain cereals, dark lettuces, bean burritos and vegetable soups. Both diets contained identical amounts of total and saturated fat, protein, carbohydrate and cholesterol, and calories were carefully controlled.

After a month, both groups had lower cholesterol. The conventional diet lowered LDL cholesterol by an average of 4.6%; the other, which followed American Heart Association guidelines, cut levels by 9.4% on average.

Fat is not brain food

A long-running and large study in California found that the fatter you are in your 40s, the greater the risk you face of developing dementia later in life. Reported in the *British Medical Journal* in early 2005, it provides the most convincing argument yet that being fat is bad for the brain.

Philip James, chairman of the International Obesity Task Force, who was not involved in the study, said it revealed yet another area of concern.

The study was conducted by the Kaiser Permanent Medical Foundation from the mid-1960s to early 1970s and involved 100,276 people who had detailed medical checks when they were in their early 40s and followed them for an average of 27 years. Between 1994 and 2003, dementia was diagnosed in 713 (0.7%) of them.

The links between dementia and obesity were measured by BMI and the thickness of skin folds under the shoulder blades and under the arms. The BMI finding was that obese people were 74% more likely to develop dementia and 35% of overweight people were likely to develop it.

The effect was stronger for women: obese women were twice as likely as those of normal weight to develop Alzheimer's disease or other types of dementia. The increase in risk for men was only 30%.

The skin-fold thickness measurements showed that there was no difference between men and women – both were up to 70% more likely to develop dementia if they had a thick fold of skin, and the thicker the fold the higher the risk.

James noted that an impressive aspect of the study was that the researchers eliminated the influence of heart disease, diabetes and all other conditions that might be the real culprit in dementia.

Why the link? The researchers could not say, but one theory is that fat cells, which are known to produce inflammatory chemicals, may cross into the brain. The quality of diet is another. Western diets are lacking in the omega-3 fatty acids found in fish and long-chain essential fats (particularly in the obese), which are known to be fundamental to brain development.

At the same time, a study led by Johns Hopkins University epidemiologist Dr Constantine Lyketsos has found that older people who stay active seem to have a better chance of warding off dementia. And it's the diversity, not the intensity, of the exercise that counts. The study tracked 3375 men and women over the age of 65 from 1992 to 2000 and found that those doing the widest variety of activities were the most likely to escape the disease.

A significant point to remember: exercising your body also exercises your brain because the brain is central to the coordination of any exercise movement. For that reason, even sitting down playing cards is helpful.

The social element

The support and help of families and friends is essential because the temptations to abandon any strict weight-loss routine are all around and within. Everyone associated with an obese person has to bolster their motivation to lose that fat and provide the barriers to back-sliding. Sympathetic understanding and encouragement, rather than belittlement, is the key.

Just why some people gain weight is a matter of much wild speculation among lay people. It is, equally, a matter of wide-ranging analysis, research and conjecture among health professionals; but all those dealing with obesity, particularly extreme obesity, have observed a startling difference between what many fat people say and the common beliefs of lay people and medical doctors.

An Italian surgeon's study of about 10,000 obese people over a 25-year period cast interesting light on the problem. Most of these people told a story of a progressive lifelong increase in weight but not one spoke of a progressive lifelong increase in food intake. The easiest explanation was that the people lied – but why would they lie to their surgeon and is it conceivable that *all* of them lied?

Other perplexing statements from obese people included: many other people (especially men) of the same age and height ate much more than they did but were still much thinner; or they didn't lose weight even when they stayed on diets; or if they did lose weight and then reverted to their previous food intake, they gained even more weight than before.

Common sense says that when many people tell the same story they are probably telling the truth, which suggests that some misunderstanding of the relationship between energy balance and bodyweight has led to mistaken evaluations and false assumptions, beliefs and expectations about the causes of obesity.

By inference, this suggests that a lot of wrong roads have been followed in the search for solutions, cures, remedies and preventives for fatness. The Italian surgeon, working from the basis that the human body, like any other natural entity, obeys physical laws, calculated that the weight gained or lost by a person with normal bodyweight is composed of two-thirds adipose tissue and one-third lean body mass and that 1kg of such weight consumes about 17 calories a day. So, if that person increases or decreases energy intake by 100 calories a day, bodyweight will eventually increase or decrease by about 6kg.

Consider that 100 calories represents

approximately the energy content of

a cappuccino.

So, how long does it take to gain or lose that 6kg? That, it seems, depends on how many calories are cumulatively needed to build a new kilogram – or how much energy is needed to demolish it. One calculation is that to gain 6kg requires a cost of 42,000 calories (or a yield of 32,000 to lose 6kg) which, on the 100 calories a day figure, suggests the total gain would be achieved in 420 days (or a loss in 320). But, since the body's expenditure of energy changes as weight is gained or lost, the time is actually lengthened to four and three years respectively.

This proposition contains many imponderables and variables. The conclusion is that, contrary to what is generally believed, the heavier you are, the easier it is to gain further weight, and this mechanism occurs with smaller and smaller increases of energy intake, so small that it becomes practically impossible to perceive them.

This phenomenon seems to explain the common clinical observation of the patient who reports a history of progressive weight gain with no progressive increase in food intake. Quite possibly, the energy intake has never altered and the weight gain has been caused by reduced physical activity, combined with the progressive loss of lean body mass which occurs with age.

One authority on obesity-related diseases regards it as probably the oldest metabolic disturbance known. Evidence of obesity has been found in Egyptian mummies and in Greek sculpture. The fact that these countries at the time were enjoying great prosperity supports the view that people become obese when society has enough food and leisure to cause an imbalance between energy intake and expenditure.

Today, this relationship between prosperity and obesity has flip-flopped. In the US low-income people, often African-American, have a greater prevalence of obesity compared with middle-income people. In US cities poor people rely on public transport and live in neighbourhoods that have no conveniently located supermarkets where they could buy vegetables, fruit and low-fat foods. On the other hand, access to McDonald's and other fast-food franchises is easy. Thus their diet tends to be fat- and calorie-laden. Temptation sits at every corner.

It is well established that obesity is becoming the norm in the American population. Ninety-eight million adult Americans weigh more than 20% above their desirable weight, and this prevalence is increasing in all the major racial groups, in both men and women, and includes younger adults aged 25 to 44. It is becoming a major risk factor for the development of diabetes, hypertension and cardiovascular disease.

Some scientific researchers believe the problem is so serious it should be attacked on a national front, through education, counselling and possible legislation, with the same intensity as the fight against cigarette smoking.

In some areas they face an even tougher battle. Early in 2004 New Zealand TV watchers were treated to – or horrified by – a documentary on Houston, Texas, the 'fat capital of the US', and apparently proud of it. Among those interviewed were people who seemed to enjoy their status as grossly obese, who boasted of being barred from some 'all you can eat for $10' restaurants because they were eating all day, without stopping, and presumably sending the owners into potential bankruptcy.

Malignant obesity is the term used to describe people 60% above their desirable weight, which corresponds to an absolute excess of at least 45kg. With this degree of obesity, there is a minimum doubling of the prevalence of all causes of early morbidity and mortality.

CHAPTER THREE

Deadly Diabetes

HAZEL DAVIES, of Eden, New South Wales, was believed to be the longest surviving diabetic in the world. She was diagnosed with the disease in 1921 and lived to reach her century.

This, perhaps, is the only good news on the diabetes front. In the US an estimated 15.7 million people have diabetes, according to official figures in 2005. Approximately one-third are unaware they have the disease. Those affected include 8.1 million women, 7.5 million men, 123,000 children under 20 years of age, 6.3 million people over 65 years of age and more than one in every 10 Mexican Indians.

Diabetes is known to affect more than 100,000 of New Zealand's four million people and may be present, but undetected, in 50,000 more – a rate of one in about 25. The incidence is highest among Maori and Pacific Islanders older than 15 (one in 12), about one in 20 among people of Asian descent and one in 33 among Europeans. Ministry of Health predictions are that the incidence is set to double in the near future.

The death rate for Maori and Pacific Islanders in the 40 to 65 age range is nearly 10 times higher than for Europeans and the forecast for the next two decades is that diabetes among those populations is expected to more than double, compared with a 50% increase among Europeans.

Australia has launched a nationwide awareness and detection campaign aimed at the half a million people thought to have undiagnosed diabetes.

The cost of diabetes is horrific. In the US in 1996, when it was the seventh leading cause of death (193,140 victims), it is estimated to have cost $US44 billion in direct medical bills and $US54 billion indirectly, through loss of work, disability, loss of life and so on.

More than 100 camps have been established in the US, Australia and Canada to give diabetic children the chance to enjoy outdoor holidays under controlled conditions – and to give their families a break from the hardships involved in caring for them.

The way we now choose to live is actually encouraging the onset of diabetes among all age groups but tens of thousands of people still don't realise they have it nor do they realise its possible consequences.

The most common type of diabetes, type 2, is often controllable through a healthy diet and regular physical activity but, if it is not controlled, it can lead to serious complications and, eventually, death.

A study reported by New Zealand's *Consumer* magazine in November 2000 concluded that for every added kilogram in excess weight, the risk of diabetes rises by about 9%.

Diabetes is directly associated with lack of physical activity, obesity and a diet high in animal fats and, with the double phenomenon of the couch potato and the newer mouse potato, the scene has been set for an alarming growth rate. Type 2 was once called 'late-onset' diabetes but now touches all age groups, including overweight teenagers and children.

Left to its own devices, type 2 diabetes can be thoroughly nasty. It escalates the risk of heart disease and stroke at a dramatic rate, it has been identified as the main cause of non-inherited blindness and kidney failure, it can damage the gums and teeth and lead to foot infection, which can become so serious that the only remedy is amputation.

Type 1 diabetes, for which regular insulin injections are needed, hits suddenly and most commonly affects children and adults under the age of 35. But it is a fairly rare condition compared with type 2.

The deadly reality behind these unpleasant facts and figures is that, once the damage has been done, there is no cure. The good news is that it can be prevented, it can be treated to keep it under control if it is detected in time, and the complications can be minimised. The risk of developing type 2 diabetes can be reduced by 50 to 75% by controlling obesity and 30 to 50% by increasing physical activity. The key is self-education and self-management, with the support of health professionals.

So how does it happen? Quite simply, it stems from a metabolic disorder, the way your body uses digested food. Much of what we eat is broken down by our digestive juices into glucose, a simple sugar that is our main source of energy. The glucose passes into the bloodstream and becomes available for the body cells to use for growth and energy. Excess is stored as glycogen (strings of glucose molecules linked together) in muscle and the liver and, when these stores are filled, it is converted to fat and stored in adipose tissue.

Insulin is needed to allow glucose to enter the tissues to enable these processes to take place. Insulin is a hormone produced by the pancreas, and the process is normally automatic, producing just as much insulin as is needed.

If you have diabetes, the pancreas does not produce enough insulin (type 1) or the body cells do not respond as readily to the insulin that is produced (type 2). The result is that glucose builds up in the bloodstream, overflows into the urine and passes out of the body, robbing the body of its main source of fuel but, more importantly, ultimately causing damage to small blood vessels, seriously affecting the kidney, the brain, eyesight and the extremities of the body (hands and feet). This may seem strange, since the blood will contain large amounts of sugar, but the problem is that it cannot transfer from the blood into the cells. Type 2 diabetes is diagnosed by a glucose-tolerance test in which the clearance of glucose from the blood is

Diabetes risk factors

Take this test now. Circle the numbers next to each statement that is true for you and then add your score.

Lifestyle

I am overweight for my height	3
I do less than 30 minutes of physical activity a day	3
I often eat foods high in fat	3

Family and origin

There is diabetes in my family	3
I have had a large baby weighing more than 4kg or I have had gestational diabetes or high blood sugars during pregnancy	6
I am of Maori, Pacific Island, Asian or Middle-Eastern descent	3

Age

I am between 45 and 64 years of age	1
I am over 65 years of age	3

If your total is more than six points, you are at risk of developing type 2 diabetes. Ask your doctor for a finger-prick test, for blood glucose, which will show whether you need further testing.

measured following a standard glucose drink given to the patient. This test may be normal in a patient with insulin resistance because their pancreas responds by releasing more insulin, leading ultimately to 'pancreatic fatigue'. Diabetes is diagnosed when insulin shots or drugs that enhance insulin action are required.

The pulmonary research group next to Peter's laboratory has recently discovered yet another risk factor: that diabetics with no symptoms of organ damage have significantly reduced lung-diffusing capacity. The capacity depends upon the capillary network of the lung, which, because of the reserve capacity of the lung, is normally not noticeable.

Let's consider another aspect of the differences between type 1 and type 2 diabetes. Type 1 patients usually have inherited immune-system deficiencies which, triggered by a virus or some similar event, kill the insulin-producing cells in the pancreas. Fortunately, this is unlikely to go undiagnosed; but without daily insulin injections, sufferers will lapse into a life-threatening coma.

People with type 2 in some cases also have a genetic predisposition but the disease is typically triggered by a lack of physical activity and obesity (85% of type 2 people are obese).

Type 2 symptoms are often mild and can be confused with all sorts of other minor discomforts. Studies in Western Australia and Wisconsin have shown that, on average, type 2 diabetes has been present for seven years before diagnosis.

What this means, of course, is that complications may already have set in. One in five new patients is found to have eyesight problems; others have numbed or ulcerated feet. And you cannot decide to just put up with type 2 diabetes. It cannot be ignored in the fond hope that it will go away. It won't.

Diabetes management plan

People with diabetes must have a management plan for the rest of their lives. As well as diet, exercise and, possibly, medication, this could involve regular self-testing of their blood-sugar levels and keeping a record of the results, according to what the medical professionals advise.

The testing is simple. You prick your finger with a lancet to get a drop of blood for testing in a meter. People on insulin must test several times a day but, if you are not on any medication, fewer tests may be necessary. But it is a strict regime so it is far better to do everything and anything you can to avoid having to become a slave to it.

The best normal blood-sugar level is on the high side of 4–6 mmol/l and diet and physical activity are critical to attaining and maintaining this level.

Diet and exercise

The best time to exercise is before breakfast when insulin levels are low and both liver and muscle glycogen stores are filled. Both weight-training (or resistance-training) and aerobic exercise enhance the capacity of muscle to take up and metabolise glucose.

A healthy diet does not mean special food. It means cutting down on fat, especially the saturated fat in potato chips, takeaways (fish and chips particularly), cream, coconut cream, fatty meats, pies and pastries. It means using less fat in cooking, cutting fat and skin from meat and chicken before cooking, buying leaner meats, choosing low-fat dairy products and fish.

It means eating carbohydrates with every meal – fruit and vegetables, cereals and pasta – and checking their glycaemic index ratings for how they influence blood-sugar levels. The glycaemic index (see table on p. 52) is a measure of carbohydrate quality based on how quickly food raises blood-glucose (blood-sugar) levels – and is a dietary key to health. Low-GI foods, by virtue of their slow digestion and absorption qualities, produce gradual rises in blood-sugar and insulin levels, and have proven benefits for health. A dietitian can advise on this.

Stay away from sugar-laden products – jam, honey, chocolate, lollies, jelly, ice cream, cakes, biscuits, muesli bars, cordials, fizzy drinks and fruit juice. Use non-kilojoule sweeteners instead of sugar in tea or coffee as a short-term strategy (artificial sweeteners do not reduce the desire for sugar).

All this may seem like a huge bunch of sacrifices of the good things in life but the alternative could be life itself. Sugar is like an addictive drug – the more you have, the more you want. Your tastes do change and foods can become more palatable without sugar.

Hyperglycaemia and hypoglycaemia are two types of blood-sugar imbalance that can occur with diabetes.

Hyperglycaemia means your blood-sugar levels are constantly high. You may feel very tired and have infections that do not heal.

Hypoglycaemia is when your blood-sugar levels are low. It can affect people with type 2 diabetes who are on tablets or insulin but more often affects people with type 1. It can arise when you have not had enough to eat, have been more active than usual or are on medication that needs adjusting.

Aim for 30 minutes of physical activity every day for the sake of your weight and blood-sugar levels and also your heart and lungs. This does not mean running or cycling up the nearest mountain or flogging your body around a gym circuit or through an aerobics session. Walking, swimming, gardening, using the stairs instead of the lift, or leaving the car at home when you go to the local shops are all good forms of exercise. There are even things you can do sitting in an armchair – isometrics, arm- and leg-stretching movements and so on. Later in this book, we will expand on these measures.

Smoking raises the risk of diabetes and, in association with diabetes, it is absolutely fatal as it doubles the risk of heart disease. That's the diagnosis of diabetes researchers.

If your doctor puts you on medication to boost your insulin level, don't abandon the sensible eating plan or the exercise programme you have chosen.

If you are not thinking enough of your well-being to do something positive about the diabetes risk, think of the money. Diabetes will cost you dearly for the rest of your life.

- You will need to see your doctor around 13 times a year – more than twice the average.
- You will have to pay for 25 prescriptions a year instead of the average of five for non-diabetics.
- You may have to pay for regular foot checks or wait months for free treatment.
- You may have to pay for spectacles, orthotics for your shoes, fungal creams and moisturisers.
- And what about blood-test meters, lancets, meter batteries, insulin needles and pens?

It has been estimated that New Zealand diabetics face extra costs of between $1200 and $1500 a year. It would be a whole lot cheaper to do everything you can voluntarily and at little cost to ensure you never become one of them.

Opinions differ on the best diet for those with diabetes. The official party line emphasises the food–pyramid concept of a sturdy base of carbohydrates, some protein and sparing use of fats. Some cynics have referred to this as the 'feed-lot' diet designed to fatten pigs and cattle and now humans.

The alternative view is that good sources of high-fat (and cholesterol) protein, such as cheese and eggs, are not necessarily villains for most people. A physician colleague of Peter's at UT Southwestern Medical Center, Abhimanyu Garg, has found that reducing the amount of carbohydrate and substituting it with monounsaturated fats (those found in olive and canola oils) to a similar caloric content is an effective alternative to the low-fat diet and improves adherence to the diet for some patients.

He notes that the most recent position statement on nutrition from the American Diabetes Association recommends an individualised approach to diet based on the nutritional assessment and desired outcomes of each patient, taking into consideration patient preferences and their levels of hyperglycaemia and dyslipidaemia (abnormal blood lipids – elevated LDL cholesterol and triglycerides or depressed HDL (good) cholesterol or a combination of all).

Dr Garg says that to control these abnormalities, either a diet low in saturated fat and high in carbohydrates or a diet high in monoun-saturated fats can be effective. An analysis of various studies comparing these two approaches to diet therapy in patients with type 2 diabetes revealed that diets high in monounsaturated fats improve lipoprotein profiles as well as glycaemic control. There was no evidence that such a diet would cause weight gain in patients with diabetes, provided the energy intake was controlled. Therefore, a diet rich in monounsaturated fats can be advantageous for patients with type 1 or type 2 diabetes who are trying to maintain or lose weight.

We think that many people will not consult a dietitian but will attempt to follow their own eating regimens. To help them, we have included a table of a wide range of common and popular carbohydrates, grouped according to their glycaemic index rating.

The glycaemic index of carbohydrates

Include moderate to low glycaemic index foods (75% and below) in your diet; try to avoid any foods above 75%.

Foods you can eat				
30–39%	40–49%	50–59%	60–69%	70–75%
Sausages	Milk	Oranges	Grapefruit	Kiwifruit
Lentils	Chickpeas	Apples	Pumpernickel	Bulgur bread
Plums	Butter beans	Pears	bread	Jams
Glucose	Dried apricots	White beans	Orange juice	Marmalades
Barley	Kidney beans	Yoghurt	Pineapple juice	Chocolate
Soya beans	Black beans	Tomato soup	Peas	Yam
Peanuts	Peaches	Fish fingers	Spaghetti	Canned peaches
Cherries	Soy milk	Lima beans	Macaroni	Buckwheat
Dried beans	Fettucine	Mung beans	Linguine	Sweet potato
Green beans	Milk chocolate	Black-eyed peas	Bulgur	
Broccoli	Vermicelli	Ravioli, meat-	Couscous	
Brussels sprouts	All Bran	filled	Wheat kernels	
All non-root		Barley bread	Sponge cakes	
vegetables		Custard	Canned pears	
Maltese			Grapes	
			Banana bread	
			Oatbran bread	
			Mixed-grain	
			bread	
			Baked beans	

Foods you should choose to avoid				
76–79%	80–89%	90–99%	100%	Greater than 100%
Fruit cocktail	Rye bread	Swede	Corn tortilla	Tofu-based
Oatmeal biscuits	Raisins	Corn chips	Mashed potato	ice cream
Potato chips	Beetroot	Shredded wheat	White bread	Dates
	Oatmeal	Muesli		Parsnips
	Banana	Rye crispbread		French baguette
	Brown rice	Crackers		Rice
	Corn	Apricots		Baked potato
	Boiled potato			Honey
				Carrots
				Cornflakes
				Broad beans
				Millet

This table is the basis for currently popular low-GI/complex diets such as the South Beach, modified Atkins and Barry Sears' Zone diet.

Weight control based on the glycaemic value of food calls for careful attention to principles and rules.

Principle 1. The hormone insulin, released in response to a sharp rise in blood sugar following a high-glycaemic meal, causes the body to switch from a food supply mode to a food storage mode.

When insulin levels are low, fatty acids released from adipose tissue are high and the liver is geared to glucose production. The high levels of fatty acids favour their use for metabolic activities.

Principle 2. Foods that promote a slow to moderate rise in glucose and insulin after a meal are not as readily stored and increase the feeling of being satisfied with the amount eaten.

Dietary intake is affected by feelings of hunger, habit and environmental cues such as the sight and smell of appealing food. There is good evidence that appetite is stimulated by swings in blood glucose rather than a drop to a threshold level – for example, diabetics with high glucose get hungry whereas individuals on a prolonged fast often do not.

Principle 3. When the body is in starvation mode, it derives glucose from the breakdown of non-fat tissue (muscle) aided by the hormone cortisol and paradoxically tends to store ingested food.

The unfortunate consequence of this situation is that weight loss occurs at the expense of muscle rather than fat.

Principle 4. The pancreas tends to oversecrete insulin when repeatedly stimulated with carbohydrates.

Conversely, when the frequency of carbohydrates intake is reduced, pancreatic insulin production is gradually reduced.

Principle 5. Not all complex carbohydrates are the same in their rates of absorption and therefore their effect on blood glucose and insulin.

In general, the fibre content of the food and the degree of processing are important factors. Apples eaten with the skin on are more slowly absorbed and produce a lower rise in blood glucose than apple purée, which in turn is better than apple juice.

Principle 6. Simple sugars, with the exception of fructose, should be avoided where possible.

Fructose is the type of sugar in fruit and does not cause the pancreas to release insulin. It is taken up by the liver, where it is converted to glucose and stored or released into the circulation.

So, let's look at an eating plan based on these principles:

- *Eliminate* sugar totally – learn to read labels for 'concealed' sugar.
- *Avoid* carbohydrates with a high glycaemic index, such as white flour, potatoes, sweetcorn, carrots, pies and sugary desserts. If you enjoy ice cream, the real stuff is better than low-fat for glycaemic response.
- Where practicable, *do not combine* carbohydrates with fats or protein. A fat and protein meal, such as a cheese omelette or a salad that mixes varieties of meats and cheeses, should not be combined with bread, potatoes or pasta. Quiche can be made at home without the pie crust.
- Fruit *should not be combined* with a protein and fat meal. Restrict fruit intake to 20 minutes before or four hours after the meal.
- *Eat* low-fat foods where possible.
- *Have* cheese as a dessert or snack.
- *Use* herbs and spices to give interest and taste to meals.
- *Obtain carbohydrates* from low-glycaemic foods – usually those with a high fibre content such as green vegetables.

CHAPTER FOUR

The Dilemma of Diet

VOLUMES OF words are spoken and countless theories are advanced about what we should or should not eat. Undeniably, the average Westerner's dietary habits have deteriorated since we succumbed in our millions to the blandishments and persuasive advertising of fast foods. Television and the print media charm us with pictures of happy Mr and Mrs Average and their children cramming their mouths with crisp chips, chunky wedges, bottled sugar, flavouring additives and other delights which come straight from their wrappers as precooked, heat-to-eat culinary 'masterpieces'.

They are, of course, counterbalanced by the flood of dietary pills, courses and treatments, but even these tend largely to evade the real issues and concentrate on selling the notion that a few weeks of this or a course of that will turn you into Miss Universe or Charles Atlas, regardless of your shape.

The real issues are those facts we have already outlined – overweight and its dominant sibling, obesity.

New approach

It may seem a statement of the very obvious but a research project at Otago University, New Zealand, announced in October 2001, postulated that a combination of exercise and dietary changes could dramatically cut many New Zealanders' chances of getting diabetes or heart disease. The researchers claimed their work as a world first and, while it may appear to cover theories already recognised, it does strongly reinforce the argument.

What Otago did differently was to target people with insulin resistance, but otherwise healthy, who had yet to develop diabetes – that is, their glucose levels were normal. In this prediabetic state, the pancreas has to secrete more insulin to maintain glucose at normal values.

The research concluded that poor insulin sensitivity meant the body produced insulin but the insulin was not able to do its job properly. This problem could affect up to 25% of New Zealanders (around a million people) and is a major risk factor for developing diabetes.

In this four-month study of 79 people aged between 35 and 60, volunteers following exercise and diet guidelines increased their insulin sensitivity by about 20%. An additional group of 36 Maori was included in the study and showed a similar improvement.

The researchers demonstrated that, if people followed the guidelines for diet and exercise *before* they developed impaired glucose tolerance, their chances of developing diabetes and heart disease could be significantly reduced. Even if the onset of diabetes was only delayed, rather than prevented, the health benefits would be major.

The innovative study won an award at an international nutrition conference in Vienna, underscoring its significant contribution to the research on the causes and controls for diabetes and heart disease.

Heart disease is New Zealand's number one killer, as it is in many countries, but type 2 diabetes has now reached epidemic proportions, affecting up to 20% of the Maori and Pacific Island population and 6% of the rest. The Ministry of Health has estimated that, unless something is done urgently, type 2 diabetes will increase by 109% for Pacific Islanders, 90% for Maori and 39% for the rest of the population in the next 20 years. The potential strain on the health system is enormous.

The cancer factor

The contention that a healthy diet and regular exercise are key factors in staving off cancer surfaces regularly and the latest support comes from several research programmes reported in *The Scientist.*

One, in California, concluded that a low-fat, high-fibre diet along with daily exercise could slow prostate cancer cell growth. This was the first study to directly measure the effects of diet and exercise on prostate cancer cell inhibition. Two groups of healthy men, aged 38 to 74, were studied. One group of 13 were overweight men who did not have a history of eating healthily or exercising regularly; the other group included eight men who had subscribed to healthy living for 14 years or more.

Both groups were put on a strict 11-day diet and exercise programme. The diet consisted of less than 10% of calories from fat, 15 to 20% from protein and 70 to 75% from carbohydrates. Their exercise focused on walking. When serum samples were combined with prostate cancer cells in test tubes, cells from the first group showed a 30% slower growth rate compared to baseline serum samples taken before the regimen; those from the second group showed a 40% reduction. Especially for the first group, weight loss was an added benefit.

The team was surprised by how strong their finding was; more in-depth research was needed, but the implications were that prostate cancer could be slowed or even, perhaps, prevented.

They could not separate the exercise and dietary components of that study but have now begun a new clinical trial focusing on diet alone with the aim of identifying specific diets to help prevent or treat prostate cancer.

CHAPTER FIVE

Heart Disease and Stroke

MOST OF US are scared of the dreaded 'big C' but our hearts are more likely to kill us than cancer and we barely give them a thought.

In the US in 1998, cardiovascular disease killed 503,927 women and 445,692 men. Breast cancer, by contrast, took the lives of 41,737 women and all forms of cancer killed 259,467.

US health figures show an alarming trend for women compared with men. One in every five American women has some form of heart or blood-vessel disease, and 38% of those who have heart attacks die within a year (only 25% of men do). The latest death figures for the US, incidentally, show 31.4% of all deaths are from heart disease, compared with 23.3% from cancers.

Again, the upside is that between 1988 and 1998 the female death rate from coronary heart disease declined by 24.7%, from stroke by 13.2%, and from all cardiovascular diseases by 18.4%.

In New Zealand four deaths in every 10 are caused by cardiovascular disease – 40% compared with 26% who die from cancers. The coronary heart disease rate is twice as high among men as among women, and Maori and Pacific Islanders, who form a significant proportion of the population, also have a significantly higher death rate. People over the age of 65 account for 84% of coronary artery disease deaths.

The upside to these gloomy figures is that, since the heart disease death rate peaked in the late 1960s, it has been decreasing because of lowered cholesterol and blood pressure levels and the swing against smoking. But the room for improvement remains vast.

In Australia 2.8 million people (16% of the population) had heart conditions in 1995, and 41% of all 1997 deaths (29,051 people or eight every day) were from heart disease.

Again, in 1995, more than 10 million Australians had at least one of these risk factors for heart disease: tobacco smoking, physical inactivity, high blood pressure or overweight. A total of 2.2 million people had been or were being treated for at least one of these factors.

A total of 7.4 million adult Australians were overweight and 2.5 million of them were classified as obese. (The population of Australia is about 20 million.)

The cost of heart disease in Australia ranges between $A3 billion and $A4 billion a year, including some half a million hospital admissions, up to 20,000 heart surgery procedures and 40 million prescriptions of cardiovascular drugs.

In Canada 23,000 people die every year from heart attacks and the Canadian cardiovascular disease bill is about $CAN19 billion a year for medical services, hospital expenses and loss of income and productivity.

As shocking as these figures may be, they pall against the incidence of coronary heart disease in the Ukraine, Russia, Belarus and other members of the old Soviet Union. Interestingly, during the Gorbachev era, an aggressive anti-alcohol campaign was conducted. Between 1984 and 1987 there was a 25% reduction in estimated per capita alcohol consumption which was accompanied by decreases in the death rate from cardiovascular diseases of 9% for males and 6% for females.

More men than women have high blood pressure until age 55 when the percentage for women becomes higher and steadily grows – three in every five cases of heart failure in women are the result of high blood pressure, which affects more than 50% of all women over the age of 55. Plus, high blood pressure is two to three times more common among women taking oral contraceptives, especially in obese and older women.

Normal blood pressure is 120 systolic (the heart contracts) over 80 diastolic (the heart relaxes) but the systolic figure tends to rise beyond 40 years of age and high blood pressure is signalled by readings of, say, 140 over 90 to 95. However, many things can briefly affect normal blood pressure in people – just going to the doctor for that blood pressure test is one. An intake of coffee or a cigarette will bump up the reading; so will anxiety or mental stress.

Chronic elevation of blood pressure is associated with excess body fat, a sedentary lifestyle and, in some cases, a diet containing too much salt and fat.

So, keep an eye on your blood pressure. Check your resting pulse rate, too; it's a good indicator of your physical condition. The resting heart rate for young adults is around 70 beats/min, decreasing to about 60 at 60 years of age, but reduced in endurance-training people to as low as 40 to 45 beats/min.

Heart disease in women has not received attention in the past because of the low incidence of the disease before menopause. A lot depends on the risk factors for heart disease to which women, as well as men, of course, are exposed – or expose themselves: cigarette smoking, high blood pressure, high blood cholesterol, overweight, physical inactivity and diabetes. The more of those risk factors you have, the greater the chances are that you will suffer from heart disease.

Smoking has been depicted as the arch-enemy of the lungs but, in the US, smoking in women causes one and a half times as many deaths from heart disease as from lung cancer; and women smokers are two to six times more at risk of a heart attack than non-smokers. The risk rises exponentially according to how many cigarettes are smoked per day.

High blood pressure kills silently. Most people who have it don't feel sick, which is why it is important to have it checked regularly. Do-it-yourself kits are available these days and, provided the one you choose is reliable, you can maintain a watch on yourself and be alerted to any change that needs professional attention.

High blood pressure can rarely be cured but proper treatment can keep it under control. If it is not too high, you may be able to keep it stable by weight loss (if you are overweight), by regular physical activity, and by lowering your intake of alcohol, salt and sodium – an element in salt which lurks in many packaged foods. It can also help to eat more fruit and vegetables and low-fat or non-fat dairy products. Anything that supplies plenty of potassium, magnesium, fibre and calcium is good for you.

Some women develop high blood pressure during pregnancy, which can pose a threat to both mother and child. Regular prenatal checks by your doctor are vital because of the insidious nature of the problem: you can feel perfectly normal but still be at risk.

The blood pressure categories below were established for women aged 18 or older by the Joint US National Committee of Detection, Evaluation and Treatment of High Blood Pressure, 1997:*

Blood pressure categories

Category	Systolic		Diastolic
Optimal**	<120	and	<80
Normal	<130	and	<85
High-normal	130–139	or	85–89
Hypertension stage I	140–159	or	90–99
Hypertension stage 2	160–169	or	100–109
Hypertension stage 3	≥180	or	≥110

*Not taking antihypertensive drugs and not acutely ill. When systolic and diastolic pressures fall in different categories, the high category determines blood pressure status.

**Optimal blood pressure with respect to cardiovascular risk is <120/<80 mmHg. Unusually low readings should be evaluated for clinical significance.

It is recommended that all women, from about the age of 20, should have regular blood cholesterol checks, because the higher the reading the less blood gets to the heart and the more the risk of coronary heart disease increases.

The body needs cholesterol to function normally and makes enough to meet its needs. But too much saturated fat and cholesterol in the food we eat raises the level and, over a period of years, that extra cholesterol attaches to the inner arterial walls and narrows the arteries.

Cholesterol moves through the blood in parcels called lipoproteins but it comes in both good and bad grades: low-density lipoprotein (LDL) is known as 'bad' cholesterol because it contributes to cholesterol build-up in the arteries; high-density lipoprotein (HDL) is good because it helps to remove cholesterol from the blood and prevents it from creating bottlenecks.

If your cholesterol is too high, your doctor may recommend dietary changes and exercise. Medications may be needed if those measures don't work. Treatment depends largely on whether you have coronary heart disease or are fortunate enough to be free of that risk element.

Unless you have had a family member or a close friend afflicted with heart disease, it is unlikely that you will have thought much about it – and you are not alone. Heart disease actually begins early in life and normally becomes apparent only in middle age when, if you are lucky, the symptoms of an impending heart attack may provide early warning. The trouble is that, in about 40% of cases, the first symptom is a major heart attack that kills its victim.

The good news is that a great deal can be done, not only to markedly reduce the risk of serious heart disease, but by recognising the warning signs and symptoms so that you can alert your doctor.

If your doctor has told you that you are at high risk for heart disease on the basis of tests or an analysis of risk factors, you need to reduce your risk through immediate lifestyle changes. It is never too late. Nor too early.

What exactly is coronary heart disease?

Coronary heart disease (CHD) occurs as a result of the narrowing of the blood vessels supplying the heart due to a build-up of deposits or plaques, a process known as atherosclerosis. This build-up is like the gunk that accumulates in a drainpipe and slows the flow of water.

Severe narrowing leads to ischaemia (insufficient supply of blood) or, in serious cases, total occlusion, which results in tissue death beyond the blockage.

When coronary arteries are unable to supply the heart with sufficient blood to meet its need for oxygen, angina or chest pain is a common symptom. More seriously, ischaemia may trigger a life-threatening arrhythmia, such as ventricular fibrillation. When this occurs, blood flow around the body stops and the victim becomes unconscious as the brain is deprived of oxygen. Prompt use of a defibrillator is necessary to prevent death.

Complete occlusion or blockage of a coronary artery produces a heart attack, the severity of which depends on the size and location of the heart tissue that is damaged. CHD is a 'silent' disease that develops over many years, often without symptoms. The process takes place in all individuals and its presence is defined by the severity of the narrowing of the coronary vessels, which is established by coronary angiography. Because angiography is an expensive procedure involving the insertion of a catheter into the left ventricle of the heart and carries a risk of complications, it is not used unless there is good cause.

The progress of CHD is accelerated by elevated blood pressure and cholesterol, diabetes and smoking. No one is suggesting that you can outrun cholesterol; to be most effective, exercise is best coupled with an all-round lifestyle approach.

If you are fortunate, signs and symptoms will warn you to take action – get checked as soon as possible by a cardiologist.

The pain of a heart attack can feel like bad heartburn. You may also be having a heart attack if you experience one of the following symptoms:

- Feel a pressure or crushing pain in your chest, sometimes with sweating, nausea or vomiting.
- Feel pain that extends from your chest into the jaw, left arm or left shoulder.
- Feel tightness in your chest.
- Have shortness of breath for more than a couple of seconds.

The presence of heart disease greatly increases the chances of a heart attack, which for many people is often their first symptom and, in 40% of cases, their last because it results in sudden death.

Risk factors for a heart attack

- Smoking
- Diabetes
- High LDL cholesterol
- Low HDL cholesterol
- High blood pressure
- Family history of heart attack
- Atherosclerosis (hardening of the arteries)
- Lack of exercise
- Obesity
- Male sex
- High homocysteine levels
- High triglyceride levels
- Excessive mental stress
- High fibrinogen levels
- High insulin levels

Primary prevention of heart disease

Primary prevention of heart disease entails the application of lifestyle changes and testing procedures to prevent the occurrence of heart disease, whereas secondary prevention involves rehabilitation from a heart attack. Exercise is more than just improving fitness. Research has now identified multiple mechanisms by which exercise exerts a powerful protective effect:

- A reduction in the development of plaque in critical arteries due to lower levels of circulating fats.
- An increased sensitivity to insulin and lower blood pressure.
- Reduced risk of artery blockage (thrombosis) due to favourable changes in the clotting mechanism.
- Improved blood flow to the heart during exercise reduces the danger of ischaemia. The increased coronary flow results from an increased capacity of the vessels to dilate.
- Reduced occurrence of lethal ventricular arrhythmias due to adaptations of the autonomic nervous system, resulting in a slower and more regular heartbeat during rest and exercise.

Talk to your doctor about lifestyle changes and ask whether aspirin would reduce your risk of a heart attack. Aspirin can help keep your blood from forming clots that could eventually block the arteries. Inflammation plays a pivotal role in the development of atherosclerosis. New research suggests that aspirin may also be helpful in controlling these inflammatory conditions. C-reactive protein, an easily measured inflammatory marker associated with increased risk of heart disease, is lowered by aspirin and exercise.

Why is exercise so important?

Exercise strengthens both your heart muscle and the skeletal muscles used to perform the exercise. It can also help you feel more energetic, more in control of your health and help you lose weight and keep it off. Exercise is also often effective in lowering your blood pressure, reducing your cholesterol and triglyceride levels and increasing insulin sensitivity.

Long-term population studies have shown that regular physical activity of at least moderate intensity, such as brisk walking, reduces the incidence of coronary heart disease. More recently an association between exercise and increased survival following breast cancer diagnosis in women was observed by MD Holmes and colleagues in the large US Nurses' Health Study, which began in 1976. For many years, aerobic exercise involving large muscle groups, such as jogging, rowing, cycling and swimming performed continuously for 20 to 30 minutes at moderate effort, three to five days each week, was considered the most beneficial. Today we know that daily exercise for up to an hour accumulated throughout the day is effective. Many recreational pursuits provide a good challenge to skeletal muscles, the heart and circulation. The development of strength through resistance- and weight-training, in addition to improving your ability to perform aerobic exercise, has independent effects, comparable to jogging, on reducing the incidence of coronary heart disease.

Overcoming inertia

As compelling as our arguments may have been for adopting exercise and a healthy diet, most people who decide to make a change cannot seem to maintain their good intentions. If you have to make a daily decision about whether to exercise or eat sensibly, eventual failure is inevitable. Weaving exercise into your daily routine so that it becomes automatic is essential. At the time of writing in 2005, the highly successful franchise operation Curves offers women a regular 30-minute exercise routine coupled with dietary advice. The workouts, which combine aerobic and resistance exercise, are structured so that there is no waiting for a particular exercise machine. It is reminiscent of group circuit training that was popular with Universal gyms. Peter Snell's wife, Miki, attends her local Curves and enjoys the convenience of a neighbourhood location, simplicity and relaxed atmosphere.

Alcohol and heart disease

The use of alcohol is a sharp double-edged sword. It is now well documented that alcohol in moderation affords significant health benefits but, at the same time, the deleterious effects of excessive alcohol consumption take an enormous social toll. It is estimated that alcohol contributes to 100,000 deaths annually in the US, making it the third leading cause of preventable mortality, after smoking and conditions related to poor diet and sedentary lifestyle.

Among the benefits of light to moderate alcohol consumption appear to be reduced risk of coronary heart disease, ischaemic stroke (due to blockage rather than haemorrhage), gallstones, type 2 diabetes and peripheral vascular disease. These vascular benefits have also been noted in studies of alcohol consumption and dementia. In the US Cardiovascular Health Study it was found that, compared with abstention, consumption of one to six drinks weekly was associated with a lower risk of dementia and Alzheimer's disease among older adults.

These benefits are offset by the risks. With heavy alcohol use, there are no benefits but a long list of ailments – cirrhosis of the liver, pancreatitis, foetal damage, cancers of the mouth, throat, oesophagus, liver and breast, hypertension, accidents, homicide, suicide, neural degeneration, heart arrhythmias, haemorrhagic stroke and cardio-myopathy (the way alcohol induces cardiomyopathy is not clear and maybe stems from nutritional deficiencies).

CHAPTER SIX

The Ways We Age

SOME SCIENTIFIC studies of human performance have supported the value of continuing regular aerobic exercise as we get older.

For instance, a 1984 study of Masters runners revealed that heart size and oxygen uptake were greater in endurance runners (average age 54) compared with sprinters (average age 47) and both were higher than age-matched, non-running controls.

'Cardiac enlargement with increased left ventricular mass is a recognised adaptive response to intensive physical conditioning,' the research concluded. 'There have been few reports regarding cardiac hypertrophy and function in the middle-aged or older athlete.' Before echocardiology and MRIs, doctors were unable to differentiate between large diseased hearts and large endurance athlete's hearts. MRIs have established that diseased hearts have thin walls and endurance athlete's hearts have thick walls; this is especially noticeable in the left ventricle, hence the focus on 'left ventricular mass'.

The researchers studied nine male Masters track endurance-distance runners and 13 male Masters track sprinters by echocardiography, systolic time intervals and maximal treadmill stress testing, which could be classified as more than thorough.

A 10-year follow-up of the Masters distance runners showed

that aerobic capacity was unchanged if training was maintained. A small loss of lean body mass was found among Masters athletes who confined their activity to running compared with those who supplemented their running with some upper-body exercise, such as weight-training.

In a somewhat downside finding, a survey by Paul Thompson of 1423 joggers in Rhode Island of the frequency of musculoskeletal injuries related to training mileage and intensity found that 35% experienced an injury and of those running 50 miles a week the injury rate was 70% for men and 58% for women. However, another study by RS Sohn and LJ Micheli in 1985 concluded that there was no association between running at moderate levels (25 miles a week) and the development of osteoarthritis.

Long-term study

In 1999 Peter's friend Fred Kasch and his colleagues at San Diego State University released the results of a 33-year study of the effect of aerobic exercise on the ageing of the cardiovascular system. This study was being developed when Peter was tested in Fred's lab in 1965.

It had been established that increasing age affected aerobic capacity, with an average loss of 10% or more each decade, and the study aimed to determine what happened when middle-aged men maintained physical training. Fifteen men, initially aged 45 years, took part in the exercise-training programme for between 25 and 33 years. Nine serial measurements were made at rest and during maximal effort. The aerobic-training consisted of swimming, jogging, walking and cycling three or four times a week, with sessions lasting from 61 to 70 minutes at 77 to 84% of heart rate reserve.

This protracted and thorough study found there was no change in resting heart rate, blood pressure, or body-fat percentage. Minimal cardiovascular losses at maximal work included 5.8 to 6.8% in maximal oxygen uptake per decade, 25 beats in maximum heart rate and 26 beats in heart rate reserve.

From this encouraging finding, it was concluded that exercise-training has a favourable effect on ageing of the cardiovascular system in older men, resulting in minimal loss of oxygen uptake, no rise in resting blood pressure and no change in body composition.

This supported a 1987 study by Mike Pollock and his colleagues on the effect of age and training on the aerobic capacity and body composition of Masters athletes. The study took the accepted fact of deterioration with age of maximum oxygen uptake and body composition and set out to find how much of the decline was attributable to ageing and how much was affected by reduced physical activity. They used 24 Masters track athletes to evaluate the relationship of age to maintenance of training over a 10-year period.

The subjects (50 to 82 years of age) were retested after the 10 years. All had continued their aerobic-training, but only 11 were still highly competitive and continued to train at the same intensity as before. The results showed the competitive group had maintained its oxygen uptake levels while the post-competitive group showed a significant decline. Maximum heart rate had declined 7 beats/min for both groups. Body composition showed no difference between the groups but, for both, bodyweight had declined slightly (70 to 68.9kg), body-fat percentage had increased significantly (13.1 to 15.1%), and fat-free weight had decreased significantly (61 to 59kg).

Thus, when training was maintained, aerobic capacity remained unchanged over the follow-up period. Body composition changed for both groups and may have been related to ageing or the type of training performed or both.

Sohn and Micheli, in their 1985 study, looked at the effect of long-distance running on the development of osteoarthritis of the hips and knees, surveying former college and university athletes by questionnaire. The subjects were divided into two groups, one of 504 former university cross-country runners and a control group of 287 college swimmers. Follow-up periods ranged from two to 55 years, with a mean of 25 years.

In former runners there was a 2% incidence of severe pain in the hips and knees. In former swimmers, the incidence was 2.4%. Additionally, 2.1% of swimmers had eventually had a surgical procedure for relief of pain. Only 0.8% of runners eventually required surgery for osteoarthritis.

All the evidence suggested that neither heavy mileage nor the number of years of running contributed to the development of osteoarthritis.

How we assess physical abilities

This may seem a fairly straightforward topic because most of us make assessments on the relative merits of players when we watch sports events. We simply use performance as an overall guide to physical ability. And this works quite well. However, it is clear that different abilities are required for the performance of different tasks. In fact, the term 'fitness' is so broad that it requires a context: fitness for what?

Physical educators for years have referred to the five Ss – speed, strength, skill, suppleness (flexibility), stamina (endurance) – and some have added a rather devious sixth, p(s)ychology. There may be a desire to add fatness to this list but this characteristic is covered under stamina. These to a large degree remain useful terms to describe components of performance.

In the mid-1960s the epidemic of heart disease highlighted the importance of cardiovascular or aerobic fitness and there was a shift away from a strength- and agility-dominated concept of fitness. This was the era when Arthur Lydiard invented jogging, which was exported to the US courtesy of Bill Bowerman and Leo Harris of the University of Oregon. Today, fitness of heart and lungs is still important but so too are the other fitness components such as all-round muscle strength and flexibility, which enable us to enjoy a wider range of physical activities, help strengthen bones and prevent exercise-related injuries.

The quality of endurance activities lasting 20 minutes to an hour or more is dependent on the supply of oxygen to the muscles for aerobic energy production, for example, you need an increased amount of oxygen when walking and running with increasing speed. Because running and walking involve moving your entire body (as compared to activities such as cycling, rowing and rollerblading), the oxygen cost is the same for everyone, regardless of size, sex or fitness level.

The maximum amount of oxygen that can be delivered for muscular contraction (VO_{2max}) varies greatly among individuals and is determined primarily by the performance of the heart to circulate blood and therefore oxygen to the exercising muscles, where it is taken up and used to oxidise carbohydrate (glucose) and fat for energy to maintain muscle contraction. A simple test of VO_{2max} is to run an even-paced kilometre as fast as possible. If your time is 5 minutes, your speed is $60/5 = 12.9$ km/h; to work out your VO_{2max} use the formula below:

$$VO_2 = 3.163 \text{ x kpm} + 2.25$$
$$= 3.163 \text{ x } 12.9 + 2.25 = 43.0$$

A kilometre in six minutes predicts a VO_{2max} of 53ml/kg/min.

A VO_{2max} of 43ml/kg/min is the average value for a 34-year-old male, according to data published in 1981.

Oxygen utilisation is easily measured in the laboratory during a strenuous treadmill test lasting three to 10 minutes, in which the subject reaches a maximum effort. The purpose is to maximally challenge the cardiovascular system and measure the response. Cardiologists routinely do these tests to put the heart under stress. As the heart beats faster and the blood pressure rises, the oxygen requirements of the heart increase, which is met by increased blood flow through the coronary arteries. In people with severely narrowed coronaries, not enough oxygen is supplied and, in many cases, this condition (ischaemia) is revealed by changes in the electrocardiogram (ECG). Further tests, such as angiography, in which the degree of narrowing can be assessed, are conducted to determine if a procedure to widen the arteries, an angioplasty, is needed.

It should be noted here that in people with undetected heart disease the combination of high blood pressure and high heart rate can induce life-threatening arrhythmia. This is partly why physicians prescribe medications to reduce heart rate (betablockers and calcium channel blockers), blood volume (diuretics) and blood vessel dilators (ACE inhibitors).

At this point, you may be getting nervous about exercise. The paradox is that while exercise strengthens weak hearts, improves fitness and relaxes arterial blood vessels, exercise that is too demanding carries a risk of heart attack in susceptible individuals. We advocate checking with your doctor before you start an exercise programme, and be aware of the risk factors associated with atherosclerotic disease.

The effect of ageing on VO_{2max} was studied in a cross-section of sedentary males in the US in 1981 and also in a 1995 Dallas study of a large group of sedentary men and women. In both studies the age-related decrease in VO_{2max} is similar but, astonishingly, the 1995 values are diminished by about 20% in men, with women a further 25% lower. These values reflect a 15-year trend of increasing fatness and decreased activity.

An extensive study began in 1966 at the University of Texas Southwestern Medical Center in Dallas (where Peter works) on five healthy 20-year-old men who were put through a battery of tests that measured how their aerobic power – their body's ability to use oxygen – was affected by three weeks of total bedrest.

As little as three weeks' bedrest in a young person has a more harmful effect on aerobic power than 35 years of ageing, according to a longitudinal study Peter Snell and colleagues at UT Southwestern Medical Center published in 2001. It graphically illustrated the theory that if you don't use it, you are certainly going to lose it.

Thirty years later, the same men underwent similar types of cardiovascular fitness tests before and after a six-month exercise regimen. The programme, which consisted of moderate exercise – including walking, jogging or using a stationary bike for one hour, four to five times a week – turned back the clock 30 years for the five now middle-aged men. They were able to regain the cardiovascular fitness levels they had as 20-year-olds, and boosted their aerobic power by 15%.

'This study demonstrates that it's never too late to get back in shape,' said the programme leader, Dr Darren K McGuire. Age had not been kind to the men, whose weight had climbed 25% on average, their body fat had doubled, and their aerobic capacity had declined 11% over the 30 years. But a remarkable finding was that the 30 years of ageing had done less to lower the men's aerobic power than had the three weeks of bedrest in 1966.

'The type of exercise doesn't matter just as long as you do it consistently,' McGuire said, pointing out that it does not take a tremendous effort to recover and maintain substantial cardiovascular fitness.

None of the fitness-training would be considered high-intensity, and it did not include weight-training. The benefits were improved cardiovascular fitness, lowered cholesterol, improved blood pressure, reduced heart attack risk and enhanced feelings of well-being.

The study findings confirmed rather than revealed the benefits of exercise. Jogging, even for recovering heart patients, had been established as highly beneficial by noted New Zealand coach Arthur Lydiard, the 'father' of jogging, as far back as the 1950s.

Cardiac risk factors – particularly age, cholesterol, blood pressure, exercise history and smoking status – should be considered in evaluating an individual's safety for an exercise programme. Currently, there is a twofold relative risk for the occurrence of coronary artery disease for inactive men compared with their more vigorous peers.

The point here is that it is essential, before you begin an exercise regime, that you consult your medical professional, tell him or her what you want to do and be guided by their advice. We want you to feel better, not worse.

Bestselling run-for-health author Jim Fixx died while jogging at the age of 52. He mistakenly believed that exercise would protect him from his high level of blood cholesterol. Up to age 35, Fixx was an overweight smoker and no doubt already had advanced atherosclerosis. It is likely, however, that he survived more years than otherwise because of weight loss and exercise.

So Fixx taught us two things, one of them unintentionally: *that exercise can prolong life expectancy and that a failure to heed a specific physical condition is dangerous.*

The American Heart Association recommends healthy people work out for 30 minutes or longer at least three or four times a week but exercising more than five times a week for 10 to 24 minutes each session is even better.

People over 45 who have not had a physical examination in the previous two years should consult a doctor before starting a serious exercise programme. So should anyone with a serious or chronic medical condition, anyone at risk for heart disease and anyone on medication. Be wise before the event, not sorry after it.

To begin with, do you know the level of your cardiovascular fitness right now? It's an important factor in considering what you need to do to get back on the ascent of living, rather than slumping onto the descent.

If your cardiovascular fitness is low, you are in a physical health area which has been linked to a significantly higher risk of death from all causes.

What are some risk factors?
- Not incorporating exercise activities in your lifestyle.
- Watching sports rather than playing.
- Expecting too much too early from an exercise programme.
- Not making a commitment.
- Making excuses, such as not having enough time to exercise.

What could happen?
- Decreased muscle mass and difficulty in controlling weight.
- Increased risk of overloading the heart during exercise.
- Loss of physical independence in older age.
- Decreased mineral content of bone.
- Increased susceptibility to life-threatening arrhythmia of the heart.

What should you do?
Look for exercise opportunities during the day – take the stairs rather than the elevator, park the car and walk 10 minutes or more to work.

Make a commitment to accumulate at least 30 minutes of exercise on most days of the week, preferably every day. Keep a record. A record is a great disciplinarian and motivator – any gaps have a tendency to invade your conscience and stay there.

Walking and hiking are the best and easiest-to-attain exercises. Others include cycling, rollerblading, rowing and other endurance activities that are easy on the joints.

Include resistance exercises so that other muscles are exercised – sit-ups (crunches) and push-ups are easy to do at home.

Muscular endurance is an important component of fitness. Training for it strengthens tendons, ligaments and bony attachments, protecting against injury in many accident situations. It also allows you to enjoy pain-free participation in activities such as gardening, golf, skiing and other seasonal interests. Those sit-ups performed with bent knees strengthen abdominal muscles, which help to prevent lower-back problems related to pelvic tilt as you age.

Quite apart from the feeling of wellness and self-satisfaction that can be got from exercising physically while others are slumped around – it is particularly ego-building if it's pouring with rain and you're out there enjoying it – there is a wide range of beneficial effects.

So, what is exercise and why is it so important?

One of the most important effects is to increase the flow of blood to the muscles, including the heart, and this is achieved by muscular activity, which requires energy and therefore an increased supply of oxygen. A complex feedback system allows the heart to adjust its output of blood by increasing its rate and force of contraction, so that just the right amount of oxygen is delivered to the muscles. It follows that the more activities you do using more and larger muscles of the body, such as in walking, jogging, cycling, rowing and swimming, the more the blood is going to flow all through your arterial system. It will also expand the arterial system, opening up capillary beds that have ceased to function because of inactivity.

Flexing your little finger is exercise, but it won't do you any good – flex *every* muscle you've got while you still can.

That's a simple view of a complex operation. Increased blood flow actually enhances the capacity of blood vessels to dilate, including the coronary arteries. A part of the same mechanism, the level of nitric oxide in the endothelium of blood vessels is raised. The endothelium, if you haven't met it yet, is a layer of cells that lines the blood vessels, heart and lymphatic vessels. It contains the important substances that are released under certain conditions to relax the smooth-muscle lining of the blood vessels and cause dilation. Another benefit is that mild to moderate exercise, which is all we are asking you to do, also stimulates the immune system. The overstimulation of the system involved in the exercise regimes followed by athletes and triathletes can work the other way, which is why these superfit athletes are much more susceptible to viruses. They can get a lot of colds and sniffles. Take it easy and you won't.

But the exercises you adopt have to build muscular strength and endurance. If you maintain your muscle strength with resistance-training, and muscle endurance with controlled stamina-training, you will become more energetic and progressively more capable of doing those exercises. Slack off, slow down and the muscle strength and durability will gradually go. It becomes a bit of a lifetime thing but your feeling of well-being will make it worthwhile.

Joint flexibility needs to be maintained and improved, if possible, and careful attention has to be paid to body composition or fatness.

This brings us back to the questions of what to do and how much to do – the exercise dose. Think of exercise as a tonic pill – how many do you have to take and how often? The first reaction would tend to be the more the merrier but that is not necessarily so. It has been determined that exercise, ideally, should consume something like five kilocalories per kilogram of fat-free bodyweight per day. Why fat-free weight? Let us say you weigh 68kg and then balloon up to 95kg courtesy of fat tissue. If the exercise prescription was 5 kcal/kg of bodyweight, the extra 27kg amounts to 135 kcal of work to be done, which in essence represents a 'fat penalty' because the capacity to do exercise has not been enhanced by the extra weight. An overweight person would otherwise face a very high caloric target.

The table below gives examples of how the target energy expenditure may be accomplished. For example, an 81kg male or female (assuming a body-fat percentage of 20%) has a fat-free weight of 65kg, which corresponds to a caloric target of 328 kcal. Walking at 5km/h would take 67 minutes to accomplish this target compared with 45 minutes walking at 6km/h or only 24 minutes when jogging at 10 km/h (6 minutes/km).

Target kcal daily expenditure

Bodyweight (kg)	54	67.5	81	94.5
Fat-free weight (kg)*	43.5	54.5	65	76.5
Target kcal per day	218	273	325	383

* Assume 20% body fat

Exercise expenditure

Exercise	kcals per 10 minutes/kg bodyweight			
	54	67	81	94.5
Walking 5km/h	33	41	49	57
Walking 6km/h	49	61	73	85
Jogging 10km/h	89	112	134	156
Tennis	9	74	88	104
Cycling 21km/h	5	95	105	115
Swimming – slow	9	87	104	122
Swimming – fast	5	106	127	148
Dancing – ballroom	8	35	41	48
Dancing – 'twist'	6	70	83	98

Peter weighs just under 81.6kg so he needs to do 408 (326) kilocalories of exercise. Since he likes cycling, and easy-paced cycling works off 105 calories in 10 minutes, he needs 39 minutes on the bike each day.

Lifestyle has an enormous influence on how people develop. The Honolulu Heart Study, which has followed a large population of men since the late 1940s, compared Japanese men living in Japan, Honolulu and California and found that between each of those places respectively the incidence of coronary heart disease rose considerably.

This was conclusive evidence that lifestyle, along with diet, is a factor in heart disease.

The study got off the ground because the Japanese group examined lived in Nagasaki, where one of the nuclear bombs was dropped in World War II, and numerous studies relating to the effects of radiation were under way there. Among the findings was the difference between those still living there and former residents who had moved to Hawaii and the US.

In Honolulu the study also looked at the amount of walking older men (70 and over) within the group did each day. This revealed a higher premature mortality rate in those who walked less than a mile a day and evidence that, if you walk one to two miles a day – and not many people do much more than that – the improvement in early mortality is significant. The more you walk, the greater the improvement, although it is not as impressive.

But walking programmes pay off.

Right there, you have basic evidence of the value of the simplest form of exercise – an activity we can do with virtually no training or preparation. Just get out of your chair and walk.

Target heart rates

Target heart rates for a 10-second pulse count			Target heart rates for a 60-second pulse count		
Age	Low (70% max)	High (85% max)	Age	Low (70% max)	High (85% max)
20	23	28	20	138	168
30	22	27	30	132	162
40	21	26	40	126	156
50	20	24	50	120	144
60	18	23	60	108	138
70	17	21	70	102	126

How much is enough? Broadly, for the 10 to 60 minutes of the exercise period, just about any physical activity that keeps the heart rate at roughly 70 to 85% of its maximum is considered optimal. To determine what that level is for you, measure your pulse. Count for 10 seconds and multiply by six or take the whole minute, whichever suits. The best pulse points are the inner wrist or the carotid artery on the neck, using the first two fingers of one hand.

To calculate your maximum heart rate per minute, subtract your age from 220.

A more informal way to gauge the intensity of exercise is to aim for a 'talking pace', intense enough to work up a sweat but moderated so that it is possible to talk without gasping for breath. Obviously, as fitness increases, the 'talking pace' becomes faster and faster.

The sweat experts divide exercise into three general categories: aerobic, strength, and flexibility. They recommend a balanced programme using all three. You can follow such programmes at gyms and exercise clubs, with personal trainers, but this can be an expensive approach and isn't really necessary. Exercise videos can be helpful but they can also be harmful, if you are enticed into attempting the levels of effort, strength and flexibility of the demonstrators. You also need to be aware that not all personal trainers and other purveyors of physical fitness techniques are necessarily adequately qualified.

Make the most of mind and muscle

Another long-term study, which began in the 1920s, examined the lives and feelings of well people through questionnaires, psychiatric interviews and medical examination. In all, 840 people have been followed from their teens into their 80s. The latest part of the study, led by Dr George Vaillant, divided people between the ages of 60 and 80 into groups designated by the terms 'happy-well' and 'sad-sick'. Those who had died were 'prematurely dead'.

Analysis of these groups determined that seven major factors predict at age 50 what life will be like at age 80:

- Not smoking or quitting early. Those who quit before 50 were at 70 as healthy as those who never smoked. (Heavy smoking was 10 times more prevalent among the prematurely dead.)
- The ability to take life's ups and downs in your stride.
- Absence of alcohol abuse.
- Healthy weight.
- A solid marriage.

- Physical activity.
- Years of education.

People who had three or fewer of these seven factors at age 50 were three times more likely to die during the following 30 years than those who had four or more of them.

The study emphasised the 'touchy-feely' aspects of life, which probably do not come naturally and easily to many people, including New Zealanders. The four attributes vital to successful ageing were:

- Orientation to the future – the ability to anticipate, to plan and to hope.
- Gratitude, forgiveness and optimism – we need to see the glass as half-full, not half-empty.
- Empathy – the ability to imagine the world as it seems to the other person.
- The ability to reach out – we should do things *with* people, not do things *to* people or ruminate that *they* do things to *us*.

Another angle on the ageing health problem is that merely being a man can be construed as a health hazard, according to Dr West of the University of Western Sydney Men's Health Information and Research Centre.

'Statistics show that men have higher rates of cancer-related deaths, are involved in more fatal transport accidents and have a higher rate of suicide,' West says.

Men are commonly found in the riskiest jobs. 'Look at those firefighters in New York, look at almost any kind of job involving risk and you will find a high proportion of men. We're seeing men virtually sacrificing their lives on the football field for the sake of being called heroes.'

He suggests that the more 'masculine' a man is, the more vulnerable he is to disease and early death.

'Working-class men are much more at risk. They're much more likely to eat fast food and they're much less likely to visit gyms. The guys who should be in gyms are lying on the couch watching the football.'

Dr West says women's health needs are better understood than men's and subject to more open discussion. 'You won't find men standing around in a group talking about their prostate problems. It's that "she'll be right, mate" mentality that also means men report fewer illnesses or make fewer visits to the doctor.'

One of the major and often unnoticed problems that occurs with ageing is the loss of muscular endurance and strength. In most cases, it just happens without being noticed. An important consequence of this is that we tend to compensate by reducing our activity level. We tire more easily, our muscles hurt, so we do less.

Over time this diminished activity results in further decline in muscle size. Throw in a little arthritis, coupled with a decreased ability to recover from unaccustomed activity, and we are caught in the downward spiral of ageing.

Unfortunately, we are taught that this is normal. But 'normal' is neither desirable nor inevitable. Just as doctors once told us that a cholesterol level of 14 mmol/1 was normal, we do not have to accept other 'normal' results, such as not having the capacity to run a kilometre in better than five minutes at age 50.

State of mind is an important factor in the ageing process. It's another of those choices you have to make throughout your life. Do you think you are getting old? That you are old? Or do you think that you are only as old as you feel and you feel great? What thoughts race through your head when you get up in the morning and take your first look in the mirror?

Your first reaction may be 'Hell, I look old', but you don't have to accept the notion that you must 'feel old'. Most symptoms of ageing can be treated. A lot depends on your level of vanity and perhaps your ability to pay to maintain that vanity. You can have face-lifts and skin-tucks to keep you looking like a 20-year-old – though forming natural expressions may become difficult and your friends may regard you rather oddly because you suddenly look younger than your own son – but growing old gracefully doesn't have to be so drastic.

Treat your body as you would an expensive car by keeping it physically tuned up with exercise and vitamin supplements and, perhaps, judicious use of hormones and other supplements designed for that feeling of wholeness.

But don't forget your mind. Having a fit body with an unfit brain inside it is of no great value. Get yourself into activities that build self-esteem, that are satisfying, that make you feel you are still a useful and productive member of society. Volunteer work, consulting, a second career, a college course, or self-improvement classes are all options that work on your mental attitude to the mounting years.

Activities such as golf, walking, jogging, hiking, orienteering, tennis, skiing, swimming and so on are great for keeping the body in shape; but the brain needs stimuli, too. Bridge and other card games, crossword puzzles and other word games, jigsaws and reading all contribute to mental alertness. In recent years the older generations, not to be overshadowed by their juniors, have been flocking to computer classes, tackling the Internet and all the other complexities with an encouraging and enlivening enthusiasm. Genealogy, for example, has become almost a Third Age industry because the Internet has opened doors wide to the past as well as the future.

You will know, possibly, of 90-year-olds who are younger in body and spirit than many 50-year-olds. Decide to join them; even decide to be a kid. Again.

Stay active with friends, relatives and pets. People are the mirrors through which we see ourselves reflected. Focus outward and you'll lose sight of yourself and any problems you might have – or think you might have. Focus inward and your problems, real or imagined, will overwhelm you.

Minimise stress. Stress is known to affect the immune system but most stressful facets of your life in the Third Age can be eliminated simply by your decision to do so.

Think about what you eat and drink. The Third Age is the time to practise good nutrition because you should recognise that your body's needs may be different in this era. Whatever you drink now, make sure a lot of it is water.

Look your best and feel your best. Skin care, hydration, proper diet, exercise, not smoking, weight control and an enthusiasm for life will keep you glowing, and feeling and looking decades younger. As the Nike ads say, 'Just do it'.

People who age well have a low risk of disease and disease-related disability. This has been a major interest of Peter's work in cardiology and the role of exercise in the prevention of cardiovascular disease. Ageing well means maintaining high physical and mental functions, in defiance of the popular perception that the older you get, the less your mental sharpness becomes. Studies indicate that maybe 10% fit that perception but the rest stay mentally capable if they stay mentally active.

The important requirement here is that you should believe in your own abilities. Many people have doubts about their ability to exercise but it has been found that, once they have overcome that self-doubt, they just take off and do well.

As you move through life, you subject yourself to regular mental workouts through the job you do, through your leisure time and other intellectual activities. There is, however, room for depression and that's what we have to guard against.

One of Peter's colleagues, a psychologist, won a grant for studying depression and exercise. She had published some work that compared the differences between people with personal trainers at a fancy club and those who attended weekly group sessions and talked about their programmes. Her finding was that the groupies did just as well in terms of fitness and satisfaction with themselves as those with personal trainers.

At the time, she was working for an aerobics centre founded by the reputable Ken Cooper. Ken may not have been too happy with her finding that a smart fitness centre may not be necessary but it is good news for those who feel they cannot afford a fitness club.

We have talked to friends about what they think about ageing and what their ideas are about being positive and avoiding the downward spiral that can lead to depression. One of them was Murray Halberg, who unfortunately developed cancer of the large intestine and lost about 13cm of it. He followed the surgery with chemotherapy and developed diabetes as a side-effect. It wasn't easy for him but, being the tough competitive type he is, he is doing an excellent job of keeping his sugar levels right.

He has continued his involvement in the Halberg Trust, which is a fundraiser for disabled children and runs New Zealand's annual sportsperson of the year function. He's also found a new interest in the Internet.

Garth, after a spinal fusion in 1973, was told by his surgeon he had to give up any thoughts of returning to running and golf. So he ran a marathon a handful of months later and worked on bringing his golf handicap down about six strokes. And he was up and back to work a day or two after his bowel cancer operation in 1985.

What this shows is that, with the right mental approach and capability, life can continue at a good level. A lot of us are too busy or *believe* we are too busy to do that. Women are better at maintaining a good level of living than men, who often feel somewhat at sea when they retire from their jobs. Most men facing increased leisure time after retirement don't plan activities to take the place of work and this is a failure that can have serious consequences.

Seeking and accepting new challenges and learning new skills is preventive medicine of the best kind. It is important these days to be computer literate and embrace some of the technology. There are rewards for risk-taking, flexibility and innovation even at the lower levels, such as merely using your computer to keep track of your finances and family and friends' birthdays and so on.

We agree that older people have more difficulty with the technology of the computer world than, say, their grandchildren (we need teenagers to programme our mobile phones and DVD players); but we shouldn't cave in to this idea that the experience of older people is not worthwhile, because there is much more to life than technology. Mental ability is not just intelligence; it's a very strong motivation and interest in a wide range of things, whether or not they appear to have any relevance.

As always, there is a downside to this ageing business. Kim Hill, one of New Zealand radio's top interviewers, asked Peter why a 35-year-old would think that an older person's experience is any good. She was articulating a widespread age prejudice among the

30-something crowd. Unfortunately, some older people are perceived to be inflexible, dogmatic and 'living in the past', which is not necessarily always the case. Individuals' interest in new information varies and new technology may be intimidating to some. We feel much more informed and smarter now compared to when we were 25, and are still excited about learning. The reason most young scientists have an older mentor is so that they can be directed into developing new knowledge rather than wasting time on what has already been done. In the wider sense, young people don't know enough to realise what they don't know. Kim Hill was probably playing devil's advocate and giving Peter the opportunity to rebut the stereotype. See, we 'oldies' are charitable, too.

When Peter was a teenager, he thought, why should he care about academic stuff as long as he got his strokes from being able to hit a golf ball better, make the rugby team, run faster or do well at tennis? He finally figured it out and totally turned his life around.

Then there's the matter of taking care of your skin. It might not seem important but have you ever noticed the skin of someone who has spent a lifetime wreathed in clouds of cigarette smoke? It's too late for that someone to do anything about it. The only solution is to never smoke or use drugs. Garth worked for many years with a woman who chain-smoked. She insisted that she rarely inhaled – the cigarettes just stayed between her lips and the smoke from the burning end created an irremovable brown trail from her upper lip into her hair. Lung cancer killed her in her mid-60s.

Many environmental factors can affect us but we can work positively to minimise stress and avoid unnecessary conflict.

Peter takes antioxidants because it makes sense to him. The evidence that vitamins C and E and beta-carotene are useful is very persuasive. Antioxidants help to protect tissues and minimise and prevent damage to DNA, which in turn helps to prevent cancer and other conditions. We all know that the older age groups are growing exponentially all around the world and that the growth will be increasingly steep as the baby boomers come through. The interesting and disturbing factor, though, is that the 85-plus group isn't showing the same trend. This book is aimed at doing something about that.

However, increased longevity is only a minor consideration for most Third Agers. Quality of life is the important factor and this brings us into the area of the functional limitations associated with ageing. *Limiting the limitations* is one way of putting it. It's a question of being able to continue doing things for yourself rather than having to have others do them for you.

In the US more than half the people in Garth's age group, the 70-pluses, will have severe functional limitations. The percentage in New Zealand may not be that high but it could well be heading in that direction. Peter's mother lived until she was 90 and was still working in the house, doing the cooking, and driving to the local store. She was a good example of this age and it would be fantastic if we could have more people like her – the economic impact on health-care costs would be great, too. A New Zealander who recently reached 100 years of age was still driving his car – and he had a licence to do it!

Peter's wife, Miki, who was a runner and is now a competitive orienteer, offers this thought: 'Every drop of exercise adds to the pool of fitness.'

Putting it another way, giving in, of course, is a lot easier but in the long term, the easy way out of doing things can also be the fast way out of everything.

Consider these strategies for improving exercise habits:
- Control overwork and fatigue.
- Develop a regular routine of exercise at the same time each day.
- Find friends who exercise and join them.
- Write 'exercise' into your weekly schedule or diary.
- Hang shoes or equipment on a doorknob as a conscience pricker.
- Set written goals specifying type of activity, frequency and duration.
- Specify 'some' exercise, not necessarily one particular activity. Be flexible.

- Arrange a reward for goal achievement with your spouse or meaningful other.
- Self-monitor your exercise habits so any improvement can be appreciated.
- Get involved in leisure activities with physical content, such as hiking or badminton.
- Expect and note any improved sense of well-being and less tendency to depression.
- Use periodic treadmill testing for fitness assessment.
- Proclaim your intentions to family and friends. They make valuable monitors.

We are what we think

What one *expects* to happen has a strong tendency to take place. The stronger the expectation, the better the chance of its outcome. How many expectations have you had about relationships, health and finances? What, if any so far, were the outcomes?

What we think about every day determines what we become and it is true that there are advantages to thinking in some positive – although we would add realistic – directions. Negative thoughts on occasions may be justified but can also promote inaction and poison relationships.

Part of being successful in the Third Age is understanding how our behaviour is shaped by mental attitudes, which are strongly affected by peers, teachers, coaches, societal customs, religious leaders, family and other influences. Like it or not, we are subject to manipulation by people in authority or who have our respect.

For a shocking but perfect example, the September 11 suicide missions that destroyed the Twin Towers in New York were carried out by individuals in whom the belief had been instilled that there would be great rewards in heaven for their sacrifice on earth. Their thinking, in the context of their beliefs, was positive.

On the other side of the coin, denigration by frustrated teachers and parents can have lasting negative effects on impressionable young minds.

Your mental attitude can be adjusted by conscious thought. At some time in their lives (usually around the New Year), just about everyone makes a resolution to be positive, optimistic, sympathetic, get more exercise, lose weight, or anything that may be considered desirable. More often than not, these resolutions do not last more than a few weeks.

The reason for this is that the real power of the mind lies in the subconscious. Understanding how to control your mental states and focus your attention on what you really want are key factors in becoming a peak performer in sport, business and in life. It depends on what you really want.

Extreme examples of subconscious effects on our lives are those with phobias – fear of flying (aerophobia), of spiders (arachnophobia), of confined spaces (claustrophobia), of heights (acrophobia), of growing old (gerascophobia) . . . the list goes on. When the imagination and the intellect are in conflict, the imagination tends always to win.

Peter's older daughter is reluctant to fly. Even though she is aware that the chances of dying in a car are greater than in an aircraft, the powerful images of an aircraft disaster override reality. Peter cannot deal with heights where a false move would result in death and he experiences a distinct physical reaction – cold sweaty palms and feet. His imagining of the consequences of falling overpowers his faith in his balance. And yet, in many other activities, he is considered a risk-taker.

Obviously, a rational approach to risks and consequences is helpful for survival and some of the idiots on the highway are testament to that.

Garth considers himself a cautious driver. He takes care because, as a journalist, he had too many encounters with the statistics of road accidents to want to become one of them. So he is always conscious of what might be coming round the next bend. Yet he cheerfully hits 60km/h-plus downhill on a bicycle with mere millimetres of contact with the road through thin, rubber racing tyres. He is not sure how, at 80 years of age, he should be classified because of this apparent contradiction. One of the idiots, perhaps?

How then can we work on changing our subconscious to our advantage? Advertising is an example of an attempt to instil information into the subconscious mind. Ads often employ the inefficient technique of repetition – that is, if you hear or see the message enough it might stick. It might also mean you never buy that product again. Advertisers also know that, if the message is delivered by a respected figure, it has a better chance of acceptance into the subconscious. (Good income is also provided to the respected figures.)

The subconscious can be modified in the following ways, ranked from the least to the most effective:

- Repetition
- Identification with group or parent
- Ideas presented by authority figures
- Intense emotion
- Hypnosis

The effectiveness of hypnosis has led to many clinical applications, primarily in extinguishing negative behaviours such as smoking, eating disorders and some of the phobias mentioned above.

Worthy of attention is the next best on the list, intense emotion. This is the technique employed by charismatic preachers and leaders, for both good and evil. However, an example that probably has touched all of us is the effect of words exchanged in the heat of domestic conflict. An insult to a spouse under intense emotion is going to stick in the subconscious of the offended and lie in wait for an opportunity to re-emerge.

Mental imagery has been widely used to enhance performance on the sports field, both in training and competition. When the going got tough in training and the urge to quit was strong, Peter found that it helped to think of a disabled person, who would have been glad to trade a dysfunctional leg for one of his that was protesting. In Murray Halberg's epic 5000 metres win in the 1960 Rome Olympics, his dramatic burst to open a 15-metre lead with two laps to go had been mentally rehearsed for days. Watch the routine of the top golfer – he visualises every shot and how he will play it to achieve the outcome he wants before he steps up to the ball and hits it.

Mental attitude has a huge impact on motivation. In theoretical terms, the level of motivation to perform a task is affected by the difficulty in relation to the recognition or reward. Thus motivation is low when the chance of success is low, even though the recognition may be high; and likewise, when the chance of success is high, usually the recognition or reward is low. It turns out that motivation is high when there is a moderate chance of success combined with a moderate reward.

Some of what we are depends on our personality. Extroverts function best at a high level of arousal and will tend to be positive, upbeat and enjoy social settings. Introverts, on the other hand, are not necessarily negative, but function best at a lower level of arousal and, in order to do this, may often appear to be 'tuning out'.

A football coach wishing to get the best out of his or her players should recognise that different types of pep talks are needed for different personalities and for different tasks. In some cases coaches need to exert a calming influence to enhance performance in tasks requiring skill and precision. You would hardly hype up someone getting ready for a chess match.

Some individuals use negative thinking as a strategy to avoid disappointment but this runs the risk of becoming self-fulfilling prophecies.

Many people feel that New Zealanders, in the spirit of our egalitarian society, tend to discourage individuals who have high expectations of their achievement potential. There is even a couple of names for this attitude: tall-poppy syndrome or, more graphically, the great Kiwi clobbering machine.

This syndrome has been attributed to envy or jealousy. Possibly, aware of their own shortcomings, the knockers look for, and point out, the shortcomings they perceive – or want to believe exist – in the successful.

This may have a lot to do with the fact that New Zealand has only four million people, so celebrities, whether in sport, television, on stage or in politics, tend to stand out. Also, the New Zealand media are noticeably quick to pounce on the flaws and foibles of the nation's 'star' performers. Whether it is fact-based or a flight of denigrating fancy often doesn't seem to matter. It is said that there is safety in numbers and New Zealand doesn't have sufficient numbers among which the picked-upon, overexposed celebrities can hide.

Let's go and take some exercise with the resolve to persevere and profit.

CHAPTER SEVEN

Fitness

Cornerstones of fitness

There are four cornerstones, a quartet of building blocks, on which fitness is constructed and maintained:

Strength

Endurance

Flexibility

Balance

Strength

In 1990 nutritionist Carol Ireton-Jones and Peter presented a study to an American Heart Association scientific meeting in which they showed that during moderate weight loss resistance-training prevented the decrease in metabolic rate often observed when people diet. They were testing the claims made in a popular book, *The Nautilus Diet*, by Ellington Darden, PhD, a well-educated bodybuilder, and actually used his weight-training programme, which emphasised heavy loads performed slowly, during both raising and lowering (concentric and eccentric contractions) exercises.

During a conversation, Dr Darden made a statement which, at the time, Peter thought was absolutely ridiculous but now makes a lot of sense. He said that heart disease develops through a lack of strength. The point he was making addressed the importance of muscle strength in exercise programmes.

In 1990, at the age of 52, Peter was still very active and did not appreciate this relationship. He did a few years later when arthritic pains, stiffness and aches emerged and he found he was doing the typical activities of lifting and carrying, working in the garden and other jobs around the house at a much easier pace.

Dr Darden's assertion that making muscles stronger allows you to expend more calories during daily activities is absolutely correct, particularly when you are over the age of 40.

When we talk about strength in a health context, we do not refer to big bulky muscles capable of lifting massive loads but the achievement of a modest amount of strength which you may remember from physical education classes – push-ups, sit-ups, pull-ups (chinning the

Human muscles

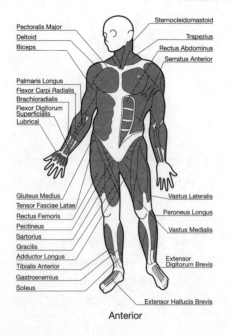

Anterior

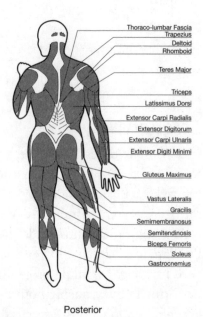

Posterior

bar) and other activities where force and power are required, such as shovelling and digging, chopping wood, rock-climbing, rowing and so on. In Peter's wellness screening of faculty and staff at UT Southwestern Medical Center, he has found that a simple test of handgrip strength correlates with measures of strength in other muscle groups.

In all of this, keep in mind that the heart is no more than another muscle among the many you have to look after. And here they are.

There are two basic types of muscle fibre classified according to their contractile properties. Slow contracting fibres, known as slow-twitch or red fibres, due to the presence of an oxygen-storing protein, myoglobin, are adapted for endurance and are found most abundantly in postural muscles and in the flight muscles of migrating birds. Fast contracting or fast-twitch fibres are white, due to the absence of myo-globin, and are larger in diameter than slow-twitch fibres. These are the fibres responsible for movements involving strength and power.

Love those muscles

A muscle is described in the *Concise Oxford Dictionary* as 'a fibrous tissue with the ability to contract, producing movement in or maintaining the position of an animal body'. That is the simple description of an extraordinary piece of engineering.

You will be aware that they exist all over you, in various shapes, sizes and states of usefulness, from the gigantic but possibly muscle-bound bulges of the bodybuilding addict to the hard-to-see stringiness of the feeble and frail – and some of our distance runners. Some structures can be worked all day without effort, compared to those which are aching and spent within an instant of extra pressure being applied.

We do all our thinking and other activities within the limits of our musculoskeletal system, so we cannot get along without making a conscious effort to keep it in good working order. The bones provide the posture and structural support for the body; the muscles, by contraction, provide the ability to move it. Together, they hold and protect the body's internal organs.

To function properly, the bones have to be joined together and the connections are made mainly by ligaments, with help from the muscles. Muscles are attached to the bones by tendons. And muscles are unique – no other internal force can make your body move – and they have a remarkable array of purposes. There are muscles in your inner ear, in your little toe and your heart is nothing more than a muscle. But, regardless of their size and purpose, they share the same basic structure.

The whole muscle is made up of many strands of tissue, called fascicles. Each fascicle is composed of bundles of muscle fibres called fasciculi. Each of these, in turn, consists of tens of thousands of thread-like myofibrils, which can contract, relax and elongate. In their turn, each of these myofibrils contains millions of bands, laid end to end, called sarcomeres – we are talking very, very small here and getting smaller because each sarcomere is made up of overlapping thick and thin filaments called myofilaments, which are composed of contractile proteins, primarily actin and myosin.

How does that astonishing complexity get you moving? Quite simply. Nerves connect the spinal column to the muscle, and nerve and muscle meet at a neuromuscular junction. When an instruction, or electric signal, from your brain, say, to leap out of the way of that approaching cyclist, crosses the junction, it is transmitted deep inside the specific muscle fibres you need to make the leap. There, it stimulates the flow of calcium, which causes the thick and thin myofilaments to slide across one another; this causes the sarcomere to shorten, generating force. When billions of sarcomeres in the muscle shorten all at once, all the muscle fibres contract simultaneously and, whoops, you're back on the footpath in time.

Without going into too much detail, when a muscle fibre contracts, it does so completely. There is no such thing as a partially contracted muscle fibre. They cannot vary the intensity of their contraction relative to the load against which they are acting. This being so, how does the force of a contraction vary in strength from strong to weak? Simple: the fibres are recruited as they are needed to perform the task at hand. The more fibres recruited by the central nervous system, the stronger the force generated by the muscular contraction. It doesn't take a lot of muscle fibre to use the keys of the computer on which this was written; it would need plenty to smash the keyboard flat.

The energy that produces the calcium flow in muscle fibres comes from mitochondria, the parts of the muscle cell that convert glucose (blood sugar) into energy. Different types of muscles have different amounts of mitochondria. The more mitochondria in a fibre, the more energy it is able to produce.

As mentioned earlier, the fibres are categorised into 'slow-twitch fibres' and 'fast-twitch fibres'. Slow-twitch fibres are slow to contract but also very slow to fatigue; fast-twitch fibres contract quickly and come in two varieties – one type which fatigues at an intermediate rate and those which fatigue very quickly.

The slow-twitchers are slow to fatigue because they contain more mitochondria than the fast-twitchers and so are able to produce more energy; they are also smaller in diameter and have increased capillary blood flow around them, so they can deliver more oxygen and remove more waste products from the fibres than the fast-twitch varieties.

All muscles contain all three varieties in varying amounts. Muscles that need to be contracted much of the time (like the heart) have a greater number of slow-twitch fibres and they are the ones first activated when a muscle begins to contract. The others come into play if they are needed – intermediate first, then the fast-fatiguers. This sequence of recruitment is what provides the ability to execute brain commands with such fine-tuned muscle responses. It also means the fast-fatigue fibres are difficult to train because they are not activated until most of the others have been recruited.

The fast marathon runner is a classic example of slow-twitch fibres in action; the sprinter exemplifies the fast-twitch capability.

All around the muscle and its fibres are connective tissues composed of a base substance and two types of protein-based fibre. One of these supplies tensile strength and the other elasticity. The base substance acts as both a lubricant to allow fibres to slide easily over each other and as a glue to hold the fibres of the tissue together in bundles. The level of elastic connective tissue around a joint determines the range of motion in that joint. Connective tissues are made up of tendons, ligaments and the fascial sheaths that envelop or bind down the separate groups of muscles.

Since muscles can only contract to move a limb through a joint's range of motion, they work in cooperating groups and more or less in opposition to each other. When you flex your knee, your hamstring contracts and so, too, to some extent, do your calf and lower buttock muscles. Meanwhile, the quadriceps are relaxed and lengthened somewhat so as not to resist the flexion. Unflexing the knee reverses the responses.

The most commonly used muscle pairings are: pectorals and laterals, front and back shoulders, trapezius and deltoids, abdominals and lower back, left and right sides, quadriceps and hamstrings, shins and calves, biceps and triceps, and forearm flexors and extensors.

Contraction isn't necessarily a muscle shortening; it only means that tension has been generated. Muscles can contract in the following ways, which are significant to the various forms of exercise and activity involved.

Isometric contraction. A contraction in which no movement takes place because the load on the muscle exceeds the tension generated by the contraction, which occurs when you try to push or pull an immovable object.

Isotonic contraction. A contraction in which movement does take place, because the tension created by the contraction exceeds the load on the muscle. This occurs when you successfully push or pull an object.

Concentric contraction. A contraction in which the muscle shortens against an opposing load, such as lifting a weight up.

Eccentric contraction. A contraction in which the muscle increases in length as it resists a load, such as lowering in a slow, controlled fashion.

Endurance

Physical endurance for our purposes means the ability to sustain exercise of moderate and above intensity for periods of 10 minutes or more, depending on the relative intensity of the effort. Endurance implies an ability to resist fatigue during heavy work. Traditionally, it has been common practice to refer to 'cardiovascular endurance', in which the activity is limited by the amount of oxygen that can be delivered to the working muscles, and 'local muscle endurance', in which fatigue occurs due to limitation of the muscle's ability to extract oxygen from the blood and its capacity to work anaerobically (without oxygen). An example of the latter is the ability to do push-ups. When you can increase the number of push-ups from five to 10 you have improved the endurance of the muscles involved in that action. The fatigue in this case is not due to a limitation in the oxygen delivered to muscles but to the muscles' ability to use the available oxygen. It will have crossed your mind that muscular endurance for a standard task (like push-ups) will be enhanced with increases in muscular strength.

The amount of oxygen that can be delivered to the muscles is dependent upon the performance of the heart, particularly its capacity for filling during the relaxation phase (diastolic function). This is the characteristic that distinguishes trained and untrained individuals. Elite athletes develop large hearts that allow them to pump a larger amount of blood with each beat. Since maximal heart rates are similar for persons of the same age, the ability to circulate a larger volume of blood per minute depends on the stroke volume (the blood volume ejected with each beat). The volume of blood remaining in the left ventricle after the heart's contraction (systole) phase is similar in normal (non-diseased) hearts but is affected by the blood pressure, which provides resistance to the ejection of blood. In persons with high blood pressure, the heart has to work harder to push blood into the circulation and the walls of the left ventricle thicken while the chamber size decreases – both unfavourable changes.

Another factor in oxygen delivery is the amount of oxygen that can be carried per millilitre of blood. This is a function of the amount of circulating haemoglobin. Levels of haemoglobin are lower in women than in men. People living at high altitude have higher values as an adaptation to reduced atmospheric pressure and oxygen availability.

When the oxygen arrives at the exercising muscles, its rate of diffusion from blood into muscles is affected by the following factors:

■ The number of capillaries surrounding each fibre.

■ The density of mitochondria (the site where energy-releasing reactions are carried out) in the muscle cell. The greater the density, the more complete extraction from the blood. When the muscle fibre does not receive sufficient oxygen for its energy requirements, additional energy is provided by anaerobic metabolism, in which lactic acid is produced and diffused into the blood. The production of lactic acid lowers the muscle pH to a level that will quickly inhibit muscle contraction (within a minute of all-out exercise).

As we have explained, muscles are comprised of two basic fibre types, slow-twitch (ST) and fast-twitch (FT), named after their contractile properties. They differ metabolically. ST fibres use oxygen readily, are rich in mitochondria and resistant to fatigue. Muscles such as the diaphragm and those used to maintain posture are almost exclusively comprised of ST fibres. FT fibres are larger and less aerobic than ST, and fatigue rapidly. Many muscles are mixed, with the ratio of ST to FT being genetically determined.

When muscles contract, the force of the contraction is related to the number of fibres activated. ST fibres are recruited first and, as the force of contraction increases, FT fibres also contribute.

The FT fibres are subdivided into FTa and FTb on the basis of metabolic properties. With training, the anaerobic FTb fibres can gradually improve their capacity to use oxygen and become FTa. However, for this to happen, the exercise has to be hard enough for these fibres to be activated because the recruitment sequence is ST → FTa → FTb.

Why do we need to know this? So that when someone tells you easy exercise is as good as more strenuous exercise, you will know that they are talking through their hats and you will understand why. Easy exercisers never get to use FT fibres, unless they are working for long periods and exhaust the glycogen stores in their ST fibres. Don't get us wrong. Easy exercise is better than no exercise and, if harder exercise puts you off or causes injuries, then easy is great. Easy exercise is a transition from couch or mouse potato status to moderate or vigorous levels of exercise.

Researchers in Scandinavia have found that people who have diabetes tend to have a high proportion of FTb muscle fibres, which are relatively resistant to insulin. When these fibres are used and convert to FTa, their metabolic profile is improved, with an enhanced insulin sensitivity.

Isometric exercise

Where aerobic exercise emphasises endurance, isometric exercise (resistance- or strength-training) focuses on strength. Adding 10 to 20 minutes of modest strength-training, which we prefer to call resistance-training, two to three times a week is important for a balanced exercise programme. People who only exercise aerobic-ally eventually lose upper-body strength. Isometric-training builds muscle strength while burning fat, helps maintain bone density and improves digestion. It also appears to lower LDL cholesterol levels. Isometric exercise is beneficial for everyone, even people in their 90s. In fact, resistance-training assumes even more importance as you age because, after age 30, everyone undergoes a slow process of muscular erosion, which can be reduced or even reversed by adding resistance-training to an exercise programme. (Please note, people at risk for cardiovascular disease should not perform isometric exercises without checking with a doctor.)

Individuals should first select a weight that allows a maximum of eight repetitions. When 12 repetitions can be completed, a higher weight or tension that limits the individual again to eight repetitions should be used. Once 12 repetitions can be completed at maximum tension, resistance can be lowered and the number of repetitions increased to 15 to 20.

While doing these exercises, it is important to breathe slowly and rhythmically. Exhale as the movement begins; inhale when returning to the starting point. The first half of each repetition should last two seconds, and the return to the original position should last four seconds. Joints should be moved rhythmically through their full range of motion during a repetition and not locked up.

For maximum benefit, allow 48 hours between workouts for full muscle recovery.

Resistance-training equipment

Any heavy object that can be held in the hand, such as a plastic bottle filled with sand or water, can serve as a weight. Heavy rubber bands or tubing are excellent devices for resistance-training; they are inexpensive, come in various tensions, and are safer and more convenient than free weights for exercising all parts of the body. Latex bands are easier on the hands than tubing. Many inexpensive hand weights are available to help strengthen and tone the upper body. Ankle weights strengthen and tone muscles in the lower body but are not recommended for impact aerobics or jumping. Hand grips strengthen arms and are good for relieving tension. A pull-up bar can be mounted in a doorway for chin-ups and pull-ups.

Flexibility

What happens when you stretch

The stretching of a muscle fibre begins with the sarcomere, the basic unit of contraction. As it contracts, the area of overlap between the thick and thin myofilaments increases. As it stretches, this area of overlap decreases, allowing the muscle fibre to elongate. When the fibre is at its maximum resting length, with all the sarcomeres fully stretched, additional stretching places force on the surrounding connective tissue. This helps to realign any disorganised fibres in the direction of the tension and this is what helps to rehabilitate scarred tissue back to health.

There is much more to the behaviour of muscles but what we have here is probably sufficient to make you realise that your muscles are marvellous devices which control everything you do. It becomes important to look after them and keep them at a peak so that you can continue to do all those things you want to do.

An important point in any stretching you may do is this: if you want to stretch a muscle, the muscle it is paired with must be relaxed. For example, when you stretch your calf, you need to contract the shin muscles by flexing your foot but the hamstrings have to be relaxed by keeping your leg straight to contract the quadriceps.

This inhibition of opposing muscle sets is not always required, however. The normal assumption is that when you perform a sit-up the stomach muscles inhibit the contraction of the muscles in the lumbar, or lower, region of the back. In fact, the back muscles (the spinal erectors) also contract. This is one reason why sit-ups are good for strengthening the back as well as the stomach.

One of the fitness myths is that some people are innately flexible throughout their entire body. But being flexible in one area or joint – the ability to touch the toes with straight legs, for instance – does not necessarily imply that the body is equally flexible in other areas. The ability to do the front splits doesn't mean that ability also extends to side splits, even though both actions occur at the hip.

There are, in fact, various forms of flexibility, which have been grouped according to the types of activity involved in athletic-training. Those involving motion are called 'dynamic' and those which do not are 'static'. So we have 'dynamic or kinetic flexibility', which is the ability to perform movements of the muscles to bring a limb through its full range of motion in the joints; 'static-active flexibility', which is the ability to assume and maintain positions using only the opposing muscle tensions – lifting the leg and keeping it high without external support; and 'static-passive flexibility', which is the ability to assume extended positions and then maintain them using your weight, the support of your limbs or some apparatus such as a chair or barré.

Research has established that active flexibility is harder to develop than passive flexibility because it needs the passive form to assume an extended position, then the muscle strength to hold and maintain that position.

Flexibility is limited by a number of factors: the type of joint, because some are not meant to be flexible; internal resistance within a joint; lack of elasticity in muscle tissue, tendons, ligaments and the skin; the ability of a muscle to relax and contract to achieve the greatest range of movement; body temperature (you stretch better when it is a degree or two higher than normal); the temperature of the environment; the time of day (most people are more flexible in the afternoon than the morning); the stage in the recovery process of a joint or muscle that has been injured; age (pre-adolescents generally are more flexible than adults); sex (women win the flexibility stakes); the ability to perform a particular exercise; commitment; and the restrictions of clothing or equipment.

It is also believed that water affects flexibility because it contributes to increased mobility and total body relaxation.

As we age, our joints tend to become progressively less healthy than young ones and, therefore, lose their flexibility.

Muscle mass is another factor: a muscle can be so heavily developed that it interferes with the ability to take the adjacent joints through their complete range of motion. For example, large hamstrings are a barrier to full bending of the knees. Excess fatty tissue imposes another restriction.

Flexibility-training

Flexibility-training uses stretching exercises to prevent cramps, stiffness and injuries. It also ensures a wider range of motion (that is, the amount of movement a joint and muscle has). Yoga and t'ai chi – which focus on flexibility, balance and proper breathing – lower stress levels, help to reduce blood pressure and may even have beneficial effects on cholesterol levels.

Authorities now recommend performing stretching exercises for 10 to 12 minutes at least three times a week. When stretching, exhale and extend the muscles to the point of tension, not pain, and hold for 20 to 60 seconds (beginners may need to start with a five to 10-second stretch). Remember to breathe constantly while holding the stretch and inhale when returning to a relaxed position. Certain stretching exercises are particularly beneficial for the back. It is important when doing stretches that involve the back to relax the spine, to keep the lower back flush with the mat, and to work only the muscles required for changing position, usually the abdomen. It is also important to breathe evenly while stretching. Holding one's breath defeats the purpose; it causes muscle contraction and raises blood pressure.

What do we do about it?

Most flexibility work should involve exercises designed to reduce the internal resistance offered by soft connective tissues. The majority of stretching exercises attempt to accomplish this and can be performed by almost anyone, regardless of age.

With appropriate training, flexibility can, and should, be developed at all ages. This doesn't mean everyone can improve at the same rate. Obviously, the older you are, the longer it will take to get back the flexibility you once had. The older you begin working at it, the more patience and perseverance you will need. If you have maintained an exercise programme throughout your life, just keep on with it.

With ageing, changes occur in our connective tissues and our bodies gradually dehydrate to some extent. Stretching is thought to stimulate the production and retention of lubricants between the connective tissue fibres, preventing the formation of adhesions and slowing or stopping an increase in calcium deposits. Suppleness is also lost through the replacement of muscle fibre with fatty, collagenous fibres.

This does not mean you should give up trying to achieve greater flexibility, even if you are old and inflexible now. Just work harder and more carefully for longer and, regardless of your age, you will benefit.

Resistance-training must go hand in hand with flexibility-training. Forget the misconception that there has to be a trade-off between flexibility and strength. Neglecting flexibility-training in order to train for strength means you will be sacrificing flexibility – and vice versa. The two types of training actually enhance each other.

If you are doing a resistance workout, such as weightlifting, the ideal time to stretch is immediately after. Static stretching, which we discuss later, at that point not only helps flexibility but enhances the promotion of muscular development and will help to ease the level of post-exercise soreness.

After the use of weights or some other exercises to overload and fatigue your muscles, they retain a 'pump' and are somewhat shortened due mainly to the repetition of intense muscle activity. The 'pump' makes the muscle appear bigger but it is full of lactic acid (the cause of soreness) and other by-products of the vigorous exercise so the muscle's range of motion is inhibited. It is inclined to forget how to make itself as long as it should be but static stretching loosens it and jogs its memory. The stretch also helps to get rid of the lactic acid and other waste matter. The muscle will then appear visibly smaller but its true size and growth are not affected. The admirable bulge after strenuous exercise is caused by tightness, which has to be relieved.

Another aspect of strenuous workouts is that connective tissue could be damaged. It will heal in a day or two but, unless it is stretched properly, it could possibly heal at a shorter length than normal.

Strengthen what you stretch and stretch after you strengthen.

The mantra is: strengthen what you stretch and stretch after you strengthen. The reason for this is that flexibility-training on a regular basis causes connective tissues to stretch, which in turn loosens and elongates them. Weak connective tissue is more liable to be damaged due to overstretching or sudden, powerful muscular contractions.

One recommendation is to do dynamic resistance-training consisting of light dynamic exercises with weights, which means lots of repetitions but not too much weight, and isometric-training. The lifting of heavier weights, which is a more intense workout, can then follow. This technique helps to pre-exhaust the muscle and make it easier and faster to achieve the desired overload of an intense session.

If you are working on increasing or maintaining flexibility, it is vital that your strength exercises compel your muscles to take the joints through their full range of motion. Repeating movements that don't achieve this effect can cause muscles to shorten, because the nervous controls of length and tension in the muscles are set at what is repeated most strongly and frequently. Cycling, certain weightlifting techniques and push-ups are examples of these limiting activities.

Equally, it is possible for the muscles of a joint to become too flexible. There is a trade-off between flexibility and stability. As a joint becomes looser or more limber, less support is given to the joint by its surrounding muscles, which is just as bad as a level of inflexibility – both increase your risk of injury.

Once you reach the desired level of flexibility for a muscle or set of muscles and have maintained that level for a full week, you should stop any isometric exercise or stretching until some of the flexibility is lost again.

Let's stretch

Just as there are various types of flexibility, so there are different kinds of stretching. They can be dynamic (involving motion) or static (with no motion involved). Let's look at some of the things you can do to keep your body in condition.

Ballistic stretching uses the momentum of a moving body or limb in an attempt to force it beyond its normal range of motion, and involves stretching, or warming up, by bouncing into or out of a stretched position, using the stretched muscles as a spring which pulls you out of the stretched position. For example, bouncing down repeatedly to touch your toes.

This type of stretching is not considered suitable and can lead to injury because it does not allow your muscles to adjust to and relax in the stretched position.

Dynamic stretching involves moving parts of your body and gradually increasing reach and speed of movement. Controlled leg and arm swings or torso twists take you gently to the limits of your range of motion. There are no bounces or jerky movements.

These exercises should be performed in sets of eight to 12 repetitions but you stop when and if you feel tired. Continuing when you are tired will tend to decrease the range of motion and, consequently, your flexibility.

Active stretching is a static-active exercise in which you assume a position and hold it there without any support but your own muscles – such as bringing your leg up high and holding it there. This also strengthens and increases the flexibility of the opposing muscles. The 'hold' should be about 10 seconds and no more than 15 seconds.

Many forms of yoga involve active stretching.

Passive stretching, also known as static-passive stretching or relaxed stretching, involves assuming a position and holding it with some other part of your body or with the aid of a partner or apparatus. For example, bringing your leg up high and then holding it in position with your hand. The splits is an example of a passive stretch, the floor being the apparatus you use to maintain the position.

Slow, relaxed stretching is useful in relieving spasms in muscles that are healing after an injury, though you should check with your doctor first if you are experiencing any pain or discomfort.

It's also a great way to cool down after a workout to help to reduce muscle fatigue and soreness.

Static stretching is regarded by some as the same as passive stretching but it consists of stretching a muscle or muscle group to its farthest point and then holding that position without external aid.

Isometric stretching does not use motion but involves the resistance of muscle groups through contractions of the stretched muscles. It is one of the fastest ways to develop increased static-passive flexibility and is much more effective than either passive or active stretching alone. Isometric stretches also develop strength in the tensed muscles and seem to decrease the amount of pain usually associated with stretching.

The most common isometric stretches involve applying resistance manually to your own limbs, having a partner apply the resistance, or using apparatus, such as a wall or the floor. An example is to hold the ball of your foot to keep it from flexing while you use your calf muscles to try to straighten your instep so that your toes are pointed.

Get a partner to hold your leg up high while you try to force it down. A classic use of the wall is the push-the-wall calf stretch, in which you attempt the impossible task of moving the wall.

Isometric stretches are not recommended for children and adolescents whose bones are still growing. They are usually flexible enough anyway, without needing to risk tendon or connective tissue damage.

A full session of isometrics makes heavy demands on the muscles and should not be performed more than once a day or, ideally, no more than once every 36 hours.

The proper way to perform an isometric stretch is to assume the position of a passive stretch for the desired muscle; tense the stretched muscle for seven to 15 seconds against an immovable force such as a wall or the floor; then relax the muscle for at least 20 seconds.

PNF stretching (proprioceptive neuromuscular facilitation is its full description) is the fastest and most effective way known to increase static–passive flexibility. It is not really a type of stretching but combines passive stretching and isometric stretching to achieve maximum flexibility. It's a misnomer apart from being a mouthful to say. PNF was developed as a method of rehabilitating stroke victims and refers to any of several post-isometric relaxation stretching techniques in which a muscle group is passively stretched and then contracts isometrically against resistance while in the stretched position and is then passively stretched again through the resulting increased range of motion.

Usually, you need a partner to provide the resistance and take the joint passively through its range of motion but it can be performed without a partner.

Here are some of the most common PNF techniques:

The *hold-relax*: the muscle assumes the initial passive stretch, and is then isometrically contracted for seven to 15 seconds, relaxed for two or three seconds and immediately subjected to a passive stretch, which is held for 10 to 15 seconds. A 20-second rest should follow.

The *hold-relax-contract*: this involves performing two isometric contractions, first of the muscles that cause a movement to occur (the agonists) then of the muscles that act in opposition to them (the antagonists). The first part is similar to the previous action but, when it is relaxed after the contraction, the antagonists immediately perform a seven- to 15-second contraction. Again, a 20-second rest follows.

The *hold-relax-swing*: this technique actually involves the use of dynamic or ballistic stretches in conjunction with static and isometric stretches and is *so very risky* that it is used by only the most advanced of athletes who have achieved a high level of control over their muscle stretch reflex.

Note that in the *hold-relax-contract* exercise there is no final passive stretch because this is replaced by the antagonist contraction. It is considered that this PNF technique is less likely to result in torn muscle tissue and is therefore one of the safest to perform.

Unless you are a professional athlete or dancer, you probably have no business attempting the dynamic and ballistic PNF techniques and even the professionals need the guidance of a coach or training advisor.

Like isometric stretching, PNF stretching is not for children and people whose bones are still growing. And once a day or, preferably, once every 36 hours is enough.

The initial recommended procedure for PNF stretching is to perform the desired technique three to five times for a given muscle group, resting 20 seconds between each repetition, although a 1987 study suggested that a number of repetitions is not necessarily any more effective than performing the technique only once. In a way, it comes down to a question of time: how much do you want to devote?

The gains of stretching

So what does stretching do for you? Here are the benefits:

- Enhanced physical fitness.
- Enhanced ability to learn and perform skilled movements.
- Increased mental and physical relaxation.
- Enhanced development of body awareness.
- Reduced risk of injury to joints, muscles and tendons.
- Reduced muscular soreness.
- Reduced muscular tension.
- Increased suppleness due to stimulation of chemicals that lubricate connective tissues.
- Reduced severity of painful menstruation.

There are some potential negatives of stretching. When performed too vigorously on muscles that have not been warmed up, particularly on a cold day, microscopic tearing of connective tissue can occur. This can result in swelling, pain and reduced function.

Balance

Balance is related to strength, agility and flexibility. As the human body ages, problems may develop in one or more sensory or motor control systems. Human beings keep their balance when nerve signals from three different systems are accurately sent to and processed by the brain. This information is then used to make corrective adjustments, chiefly by the muscles that maintain posture. Weak muscles and ankle joints are common reasons for poor balance.

On the sensory side, the systems are the eyes (vision), pressure sensors in the legs and torso (proprioception), and inner-ear balance organs (vestibular system). To help overcome balance problems due to impaired vestibular function, the brain needs to receive added information from the visual and proprioceptive systems. The more signals the brain receives from the two remaining systems, the better the balance will be. Here are some suggestions for improving signal strength and interaction from vision and proprioception (muscles) systems:

- Use your eyes as much as possible.
- Place nightlights in bedrooms, halls and bathrooms.
- Train your leg muscles by exercising on a variety of uneven surfaces (grass, sand, trails, hills, etc.).
- Increase your muscle strength with exercise and sports activity, e.g., orienteering, which can be done at your own pace.
- Do balance exercises. Stand on one leg with eyes open and closed. Use the back of a chair for support initially if necessary.
- Walk a straight line. Make it difficult by walking on a log or a piece of timber. Near his home, Peter uses an abandoned railway, which is perfect.
- When it is dark, use a flashlight. Try running on a golf course at night (as Peter once did at Chamberlain Park, a golf course in Auckland) to see how difficult it is without good vision.

Good balance can be a lifesaver in the prevention of falls, the most common reason for emergency room visits by people over the age of 65.

The cornerstones of fitness sounds simple when expressed in just these four words and, in fact, their achievement can also be simple if you're prepared to commit to an easy regimen of exercise, to persevere with a programme and resist any temptation to become a fitness addict.

We mention the addiction risk because Sport and Recreation New Zealand (SPARC), which used to be called the Hillary Commission, has suggested that some people overcompensate for working long hours by running too far, pumping too much iron or training too long. They're the opposite of those who feel so exhausted when they get home from work, they never leave the couch. Neither extreme is a healthy preoccupation and our aim is to comfortably ease you in somewhere between the two by explaining just what is a healthy amount of exercise.

SPARC spokesman John Boyd advanced the simple guideline that everyone could or should do 30 minutes of moderate exercise a day, which is not a bad starting point and it has all kinds of variables that make it possible to get your fitness kicks without specific constraints of time and place.

SPARC conducted a study in 2005 which showed that walking topped the list of 10 physical activities most likely to get people up and moving – it was chosen by 80% of women and 59% of men questioned in the study. That's fine but SPARC is more concerned with those who don't run or jump or swim or do anything else that stimulates their bodies.

And so are we. Boyd's solution is what he ingeniously calls 'snack-tivity'. This involves snacking on exercise – using short bursts of activity that add up to the magic 30 minutes. This could involve getting off the bus a stop or two early and walking the rest, mowing the lawn, or leaving the car in the garage when a trip to the nearby shop is required. Even busy people can do it. Quite easily, it can become part of the daily routine. This is sound advice in an era where more and more people in the younger age groups are either exercise 'junkies' or opt to hire other people to do all the household chores that their parents and grandparents did as a matter of course.

Boyd's problem is that many people who begin to see the results of their exercising start to become compulsive, wanting to see results more and more quickly. These are the 'junkies' or 'fitness freaks' and some medical opinion is that they are risking the start of overtraining syndrome. This can cause disturbing mood swings, elevated pulse rate and blood pressure while resting, greater susceptibility to infection, overuse injuries to soft tissues, an inexplicable decline in physical performance, and occasional nausea and insomnia.

Young women who ride the exercise bandwagon too strenuously may have problems with their menstrual cycle. They become susceptible to osteoporosis because, if they shed *too much* fat and stop menstruating, they risk losing the oestrogen needed to build bones.

Overexercising also stresses the body and this, in turn, can decrease the efficiency of the immune system. Overuse can lead to stress fractures, osteoarthritis and knee, hip and feet problems.

Under the thoughtfully provocative headline 'Hoof it', *New Zealand Listener* magazine health writer Noel O'Hare told his readers in October 2001 that they have two doctors they should consult regularly – their left leg and their right leg.

He wrote: 'If I could afford it, I would not own a car. If I could afford it, I would travel on foot. Unfortunately, like most people, walking everywhere is beyond my means: I am time-poor.

'The health benefits of walking are well known. It reduces the risk of heart disease, breast cancer, diabetes, colon cancer and stroke. A brisk 3km walk can reduce the risk of impotence by improving blood flow through the blood vessels. Walking maintains weight loss, alleviates lower back pain and increases muscular strength, relieves stress and helps to lift depression.'

O'Hare borrowed from the English historian GM Trevelyan (1876–1962), who wrote: 'I have two doctors, my left leg and my right. When body and mind are out of gear (and those twin parts of me live at such close quarters that one always catches the melancholy from the other), I know I shall only have to call in my doctors and I shall be well again.'

In her book, *Wanderlust: A History of Walking*, Rebecca Solnit pinpoints walking as the defining characteristic of human development: 'It is a state in which the mind, the body and the world are aligned, as though there were three characters finally in conversation together, three notes suddenly making a chord. Walking allows us to be in our bodies and in the world without being made busy by them. It leaves us free to think without being wholly lost in our thoughts.'

Many people, she argues, now live in a series of interiors – home, car, gym, office, shops, disconnected from each other (we would add: by the shortest possible distances in most instances).

'On foot, everything stays connected, for while walking one occupies the spaces between these interiors. One lives in the whole world rather than in interiors built up against it.'

O'Hare adds another lure to the attraction of walking by pointing out that when you walk you take part in a great human tradition. The Greek philosophers, for example, were known as the Peripatetic School (peripatetic meaning 'going from place to place'). For many, walking has been a great aid to thought – and has been practised by philosophers from Jean-Jacques Rousseau to Thomas Hobbes, who had an inkhorn built into his walking stick so he could jot down notes as he went along.

O'Hare describes the poet William Wordsworth as one of history's great walkers, having traversed a distance of 175,000 to 180,000 English miles, according to Thomas De Quincey. Wordsworth composed poetry as he walked – the rhythm of his walking can be detected in one of his best poems, *Tintern Abbey*.

But O'Hare concedes that it's no longer possible to walk everywhere we need to go, even if we had the time. 'In a sense, the car has become a prosthetic, and though prosthetics are usually for injured and missing limbs, the auto-prosthetic is for a conceptually impaired body or a body impaired by the creation of a world that is no longer human in scale.'

He quotes Solnit again: 'The body that used to have the status of a work animal now has the status of a pet: it does not provide real transport, as a horse might have; instead the body is exercised as one might a dog.'

Bizarrely, Solnit says, this exercise often takes place in factory-like gyms where people use treadmills, 'a device with which to go nowhere in places where there is nowhere to go'.

Gyms are used to build muscles that may not be useful or used for any practical purpose. 'Efficiency in exercise means that consumption of calories takes place at the maximum rate, exactly the opposite of what workers aim for. Exertion for work is about how the body shapes the world, exertion for exercise is about how the body shapes the body.'

O'Hare makes the cynical but accurate point that people are prepared to pay money to exercise their bodies in a gym but many are reluctant to walk any distance. The mental radius of how far they are willing to go on foot seems to be shrinking.

In defining neighbourhoods and shopping districts, planners work to what they call a mental radius of a quarter of a mile, the distance that can be walked in five minutes. But watch the cars in any supermarket jostle for the parking slots nearest the entrance and the feeling grows that, for the average shopper, the radius might be no more than 20 metres from car to building.

In some countries, and the US is one of them, walkers are regarded with suspicion in some areas or their activities are hampered by six-lane highways or lack of pavements. O'Hare comments, 'We're lucky here [in New Zealand] to have the freedom and space to walk. For health and well-being, we should make the most of it.'

So walking is perhaps the first and simplest step, if you'll pardon the painful pun. But what follows?

The guidelines for aerobic exercise published by the American College of Sports Medicine (ACSM) and the Centers for Disease Control recommend the following:

For healthy adults

Frequency: three to five times per week

Intensity: 55/65% to 90% maximum heart rate (HRmax) and/or 11 to 17 rate of perceived exertion (RPE)

Time: Continuous or accumulated activity 20 to 60 minutes each exercise day

Type: Activities that use large muscle groups in dynamic, repetitive motion

For the elderly

Frequency: three to four times per week

Intensity: 55 to 70% HRmax and/or 11 to 13 RPE

Time: Continuous or accumulated activity 20 minutes minimum each exercise day

Type: Activities that use large muscle groups in dynamic, repetitive motion

The American Heart Association says that, for health benefits to the heart, lungs and circulation, most healthy people should perform any vigorous activity for at least 30 to 60 minutes, three to four days each week at 50 to 75% of HRmax. Physical activity need not be strenuous to bring health benefits. Moderate-intensity physical activities for 30 minutes or longer on most days provide some benefits. What's important is to include activity as part of a regular routine.

The training effects of such activities are most apparent at exercise intensities that exceed 50% of a person's exercise capacity (HRmax). If you're physically active regularly for longer periods or greater intensity, you're likely to benefit more. But don't overdo it. Too much exercise can give you sore muscles and raise your risk for injury.

For people who can't exercise vigorously or who are sedentary, even moderate-intensity activities, when performed daily, can have some long-term health benefits: for example, walking for pleasure, gardening, housework, dancing, prescribed home exercise and recreational non-competitive activities such as tennis, badminton and soccer.

Playing basketball around a single hoop, one on one or two on two, can become pretty vigorous, but if the effort level is kept under sensible control, it can be an excellent workout even for the unfit.

The six-minutes-a-week workout

New findings from researchers at McMaster University in Canada suggest that just six minutes of intense exercise a week could be as effective as an hour of daily moderate activity.

'Short bouts of very intense exercise improved muscle health and performance comparable to several weeks of traditional endurance-training,' says Martin Gibala, an associate professor in the Department of Kinesiology at McMaster.

The research, which was published in the June 2005 edition of the *Journal of Applied Physiology*, found that performing repeated bouts of high-intensity 'sprint'-type exercise resulted in profound changes in skeletal muscle and endurance capacity, similar to training that requires hours of exercise each week.

The study was conducted on 16 subjects: eight who performed a two-week sprint-interval training programme and eight who did no exercise-training. The training programme consisted of between four and seven 30-second bursts of 'all out' cycling followed by four minutes of recovery three times a week for two weeks. Researchers found that endurance capacity in the sprint group increased on average from 26 to 51 minutes, whereas the control group showed no change. The muscles of the trained group also showed a significant increase in citrate synthase, an enzyme that is indicative of the tissue's ability to utilise oxygen.

'Sprint-training may offer an option for individuals who cite "lack of time" as a major impediment to fitness and conditioning,' said Gibala. 'This type of training is very demanding and requires a high level of motivation; however, less frequent, higher intensity exercise can indeed lead to improvements in health and fitness.'

How to go about it

You should develop your own routine and select your exercises to suit your lifestyle but a few simple rules should always be followed.

- Use warm-up exercises for five to 10 minutes before your workout. The older you are the longer it will take to warm your muscles. Try walking briskly, arm-swinging or jogging gently in place. Don't stretch. Stretching can injure cold muscles.
- Don't eat two hours before vigorous exercise.
- Drink plenty of water before, during and after a workout.
- Adjust activity according to the weather.
- Reduce activity when ill or fatigued.
- During exercise, listen to your body to detect any warning symptoms or signals.

- If those symptoms or signals include chest pain, irregular heartbeat, undue fatigue, nausea, unexpected breathlessness or light-headedness, consult your doctor at once.
- Warm down by walking slowly until the heartbeat is 10 to 15 beats above normal resting rate. Stopping too abruptly can sharply reduce blood pressure, a danger for older people, and cause muscle cramping. Now you can stretch because your muscles are warm. Think about specific muscles to stretch. The jogger or cyclist should emphasise the hamstrings, calves, groin and quadriceps. Swimmers should focus on the groin, shoulders and back.

What do I wear?

Americans spend nearly $US2 billion a year on home exercise equipment when about all that is really necessary for an effective workout is a good pair of shoes that are well made, well fitting, broken in but not worn down, and comfortable, loose-fitting clothing, anything from shorts when it's hot to pants and a jersey when it's cold. Designer gear is nice but strictly a non-contributor to physical well-being.

If your exercise takes you outdoors at night, you need to consider the safety aspect – light-coloured clothing and a reflective vest. Cyclists, rollerbladers and equestrians need to add helmets and other protective gear, such as elbow and knee guards, gloves and adequate front and rear lighting.

Exercise intensity

There are three ways to measure your exercise intensity, and they are all connected to your heart rate. The easiest and most efficient is to wear a heart-rate monitor, available in most sporting goods stores and also through mail order. You can also take your own pulse and count for 10 seconds. Finding your pulse and then counting it while counting the seconds on your watch can be a little tricky, but you get used to it. Refer to the target heart rate table on p. 118 to make sure you are within the ranges for your age.

Exercise recommendations for optimal ageing and prevention of disease in older adults

Dose	Resistance-training	Aerobic-training	Flexibility-training	Balance-training
Frequency	2–3 days/week	3–7 days/week	1–7 days/week	1–7 days/wk
Volume	1–3 sets of 8–12 reps 8–10 major muscle groups	20–60min per session	Major muscle groups 1 sustained stretch (20 seconds) of each	1–2 sets of 4–10 different exercises emphasising dynamic postures**
Intensity[†]	15–17 on RPE Scale (70–80% one repetition max), 1 min rest between sets	12–13 on RPE Scale (50–70% maximal heart rate)	Progressive neuromuscular facilitation technique*	Progressive difficulty as tolerated[†]
Requirements For safety and maximal efficacy	Slow speed, no ballistic movements, day of rest between sessions Good form, no substitution of muscles No breath holding Increase weight progressively to maintain relative intensity If equipment available, power-training (high-velocity, high-loading) provides benefits of increased strength and power	Low-impact activity Weight-bearing if possible, include standing or walking Increase workload progressively to maintain relative intensity	Static rather than ballistic stretching**	Safe environment or monitoring Dynamic rather than static modes Gradual increase in difficulty as competence is demonstrated

* Proprioceptive neuromuscular facilitation involves stretching as far as possible, then relaxing the involved muscles, then attempting to stretch further, and finally holding the maximal stretch position for at least 20 seconds.

** Examples of balance activities include t'ai chi movements, standing yoga or ballet movements, standing on one leg, stepping over objects, climbing up and down stairs slowly, turning, standing on heels and toes.

† Intensity is increased by decreasing the base of support (e.g., progressing from standing on two feet while holding the back of a chair to standing on one foot with no hand support); by decreasing other sensory input (e.g., closing eyes or standing on a foam pillow); or perturbing the centre of mass (e.g., holding a heavy object out to one side while maintaining balance, standing on one leg while lifting the other to different positions).

Target heart rate table

Target heart rate (THR) determined by the intensity of the workout and your maximum heart rate (MHR).

Age	Low intensity* (beats/min) 50–60% of MHR	Moderate intensity* (beats/min) 60–75% of MHR	High intensity* (beats/min) 75–85% of MHR
under 20	17–20	20–25	25–28
20–30	16–19	19–24	24–27
30–40	15–18	18–22	22–26
40–50	14–17	17–21	21–24
50–60	13–16	16–20	20–23
60–70	12–15	15–19	19–21
70–80	12–14	14–18	18–20

The best time to judge if you are working in the THR zone is immediately after exercising. Find your pulse at your radial (on the wrist) or carotid (side of neck) artery and count the beats per minute.

Another method involves measuring your rate of perceived exertion (RPE). This lets you rate your effort on a scale of seven to 20 (the scale being chosen in relation to the heart rate of a young person, which varies from 70 at rest to 200 at exhaustion – the RPE with a zero added) and then consult the following table to estimate your percentage of maximum heart rate. For example, if you feel you are at 14 on the RPE scale, the chart indicates 70–80% maximal heart rate, the recommended intensity for aerobic conditioning. The table also describes the 'talk test' which is a very good gauge for measuring intensity.

Judging whether you are working hard enough depends on your purpose. To train the heart and keep it healthy, the intensity can be between 60 and 85% of your maximum heart rate. A moderate intensity (70 to 75%) is more appropriate for daily weight management. If you want to win your next 5K, do 30-second intervals at 90% of maximum heart rate interspersed in your regular workout.

Rate of perceived exertion (RPE) table

Level	Heart rate	RPE	Talk test
Easy	50–60%	7–9	Talking is easy
Moderate	60–70%	10–12	You are still able to talk but it takes a little more effort
Aerobic	70–80%	13–15	Breathing is challenged and you are not inclined to chat
Threshold	80–90%	16–18	You are panting pretty hard and conversation is nearly impossible
Cut-off	90 and above	19–20	You can not sustain this intensity for more than a minute

Modified from *Fitness Magazine*, January/February 1998.

CHAPTER EIGHT

The Use It Or Lose It Exercise Programme

Each day

Morning
- 15 minutes warm-up strengthening and gentle flexibility exercises.
- 20 to 30 minutes aerobic exercise at moderate effort, approximately 75% maximal heart rate.
- 5 minutes stretching post–exercise.

Afternoon or evening
On alternate days do 20 to 30 minutes aerobic exercise (preferably a different type from the morning) and resistance-training (sample exercises).

What is an exercise stress test?

When Peter does a stress test, his purpose is to objectively assess fitness by measuring the amount of oxygen consumed during increasing levels of exercise designed to produce exhaustion in six to 10 minutes. It is now well established that low levels of fitness are a strong indicator of early mortality. A former colleague of Peter's, Dr Chris Cole, now at the Mayo Clinic, has found that prolonged elevation of the heart rate after such a test is an additional indicator of heart problems. On the other hand, moderate and above fitness is associated with a healthy cardiovascular system, which recovers quickly after exhausting exercise.

A cardiologist uses a stress test to estimate the condition of the coronary vessels that supply oxygen to the heart for its energy needs. When coronary arteries are severely narrowed, the heart may not get enough blood during heavy exercise and this is often revealed by changes in the electrocardiogram – a feature known as S–T segment depression. The work of the heart is primarily determined by the heart rate and the pressure (the systolic pressure) it must overcome to push blood into the main artery leaving the heart. Thus a weak heart is protected by drugs that lower the heart rate and blood pressure.

Once the cardiologist believes there is a problem, further tests such as echocardiography, radionuclear imaging or an angiogram may be needed to determine if angiography or other procedures are necessary.

From this discussion, you may conclude that rest and not exercise should be recommended. This seems reasonable and was for many years the way heart patients were treated. Now, of course, we know that rest will cause further deconditioning of muscles, including the heart, and reduce the chances of recovery. In chapter six we mentioned that a number of people had heart attacks or died during jogging. Further analysis shows that if 1000 people who jogged an hour a day were to have a heart attack, we would expect 41 of these to occur during the jogging activity (1/24th of their life) by random chance alone. This is not to suggest that a person over 50 years of age should not be careful or fail to be checked for 'silent' heart disease before starting an exercise programme.

Balance self-test

- Have you fallen more than once in the past year?
- Do you take medicine for two or more of the following diseases: heart disease, hypertension, arthritis, anxiety or depression?

- Do you have dizziness or balance problems frequently?
- Have you experienced a stroke or other neurological problem that has affected your balance?
- Do you experience numbness or loss of sensation in your legs and/or feet?
- Are you inactive?
- Do you feel unsteady when you are walking?

If you answered 'yes' to one or more of the above questions, you could have a balance problem. Consult your doctor.

Assess how fit you are

Your fitness can be assessed in less than five minutes with surprising accuracy. Try these tests.

Fatness. The old adage 'can you pinch an inch?' is relevant. In most men, excess weight (fat) goes on around the middle; therefore the area close to the umbilicus is predictive of body fat. If you squeeze the fat layer together to form a double fold vertically, it should be no more than 2.5cm.

In women, fat seems to accumulate on the thighs but this area is difficult to 'pinch'. A more accurate assessment is on the back of the arm over the triceps muscle with the fold parallel to the long axis of the upper arm.

Muscle strength. The tests are push-ups for upper body strength and bent-knee sit-ups for abdominal strength – muscles that for many people do not get much use. Men over 50 years should be able to do at least 10. Excess weight may limit performance.

Women are allowed to do push-ups on their knees (rather than toes).

Both men and women should be able to do at least 20 sit-ups.

Flexibility. A representative measure of flexibility is the 'sit and reach'.

While sitting on the floor with the legs straight and soles of feet against a wall, gently reach towards the toes with hands together and fingers extended. Proceed only to the point of tightness and repeat a few times. You should be able to reach your toes.

Aerobic endurance. Running on the spot for three minutes. If this leaves you breathless, it's time to do some brisk walking, or even better a combination of walking and jogging, preferably on grass or some other soft surface.

As the body ages the first requirement is to maintain muscle tone so that exercises can be sustained as we advance into our 60s, 70s, 80s and beyond. Without muscle activity, there can be no benefits to the cardiovascular, respiratory and other systems.

Often we stop activity that would maintain muscle tone because we get tired or joints ache with the beginnings of arthritis. We have to resist this temptation to quit because quitting is a direct step towards a worsening of whatever the temptation is. The more we give up, the harder it becomes to start again and get back what we surrendered in the first place.

It is essential to go for lifestyle choices that enhance energetic behaviour, such as achieving and maintaining ideal weight, getting adequate rest, taking prudent exercise (rather than being a weekend warrior) and using anti-inflammatory medications judiciously.

If muscle tone is poor at the starting point of your keep-fit regime, the exercise must be relatively simple and easy to do. The gym, however beguiling its promotional approach, should not be the first step. It can be money badly spent.

Be careful about gymnasium programmes in which you are under the control of 'fitness experts'. As Noel O'Hare suggested, demanding routines such as weights, circuits, high-speed dance routines and so on can become addictive. Participants can overstep the limits of their fitness and injure themselves trying to keep up with their peers or their instructors. These programmes may be okay for show-offs in the latest gear but most women who really need to exercise would be intimidated in these classes and would be unlikely to stay with them, even if they were getting some benefit.

Isometric exercises can be used to tone most muscle groups and they are at your fingertips, to be performed anywhere at any time:

- Push down or pull up the edge of the chair you're sitting on while reading this.
- Put one foot on the other foot and push/pull to exercise most of your leg muscles. Don't forget to swap feet over to maintain a balance.
- Stand in a doorway and push against the frame.
- Press in and pull out the steering wheel of your car while you're waiting for the lights to change or the traffic jam to move.

You can use your arms and legs inventively to oppose each other, the guiding principle being that any isometrics should be designed always to counterbalance muscle groups. If you push, you should also pull. Any exercise that causes muscles to contract is beneficial. The benefit may be local or systemic, depending on the capacity of the muscle to exert force. The benefit increases in proportion to the percentage of maximal force that is used.

For instance, you can improve the strength of the flexor muscle of the little finger using this principle but the caveat is always that exerting maximal exertion may damage unconditioned muscles and connective tissue.

Another factor is the capacity of the muscle to produce energy to sustain its activity (muscle endurance); the benefit increases in proportion to the number of times the muscle contracts.

The systemic effect kicks in when the amount of muscle activation requires increased delivery of oxygen, which improves the cardiovascular, respiratory, endocrine and immune systems. Generally, more total exercise can then be accomplished without damage or overtraining.

Two hours of walking at 3km/h burns 574 calories for an 80kg person. Jogging at 10-minute miles will expend those calories in 44 minutes. So which gives you the best bang for your calories?

The faster pace is probably better because more muscle is involved in the action so more muscle fibres receive a training stimulus.

Next question: Is two hours' repetitive contraction for any given muscle fibre as good as 44 minutes at a faster pace? That we don't know. All we do know is that both are valuable exercises and the one you choose should be the one that you prefer and, therefore, are more likely to enjoy. That's a psychological benefit.

The best exercises are the ones that you will do regularly

Exercising can be boring, which is probably why the group sociability offered by fitness centres catches on. Your motivation is helped by something more than a 'good for your health' reason but it isn't always feasible to get your exercise through organised activities such as team sports.

A wide range of stomach crunches, sit-ups, press-ups and so on, with varying degrees of difficulty, can be adopted without leaving home. For example, if you can't manage the traditional press-up on hands and toes, do them with your knees on the floor. In time, you'll be up on your toes. Look particularly for exercises that help to prevent back problems, a major source of disability, and avoid any that might make a bad back condition worse.

How long should a muscle contraction be maintained to gain maximum benefit? How many times should a specific contraction be used in an exercise session? Which is best: one-second contractions in sets of six or seven; seven-second contractions in sets of three or four; or 20-second contractions with 20-second rests three times?

How often should you exercise? Once a day? Once every 36 hours? Three, four or seven times a week? For 15 minutes or half an hour at a time? Or longer?

What degree of effort is most effective – 100%, 80%, 60%?

The fitness experts – and there are more of them than you can count – vary widely in their answers to these questions. Many of their traditional beliefs become entrenched and remain there until research challenges them – and even the research can be controversial.

For instance, one school of thought recommends thorough stretching before any exercise is started. So people contort themselves against fences and power poles before going running or jogging, not appreciating that stretching cold muscles can mean the run or jog won't even start. The pre-run stretch can do more harm than good.

Another school of thought recommends gentle jogging to warm up, with any stretching to follow after the exercise has been completed. This is the school to enrol in because muscles need to be warm before they are stretched and the stretching should never cause discomfort. It should always be gentle. So pre-activity stretching is a no-no.

As a runner, Peter found calf-muscle stretching was more effective if he exercised and warmed the calf with rhythmical heel-lifts for a minute or two and then stretched.

Assuming we have achieved a level of muscle tone that enables regular exercise to be undertaken, where do such aids as exercycles, stationary bicycles, rowing machines, treadmills and so on fit in? They target different muscle groups and, ideally, we should exercise as many muscles of the body as we can. The rowing machine is good because it works back and arm muscles as well as leg muscles. But all have similar beneficial effects on the heart and circulation. Some people may be able to achieve greater caloric expenditure on a treadmill than on an exercycle. Exercycles come in a range of wheel weights, tension controls and resistance pads and, ideally, should always pose something of a challenge to the user.

The choice, again, is yours. Our only injunction is that you make the choice.

Moving out of doors, think about walking, jogging, running, cycling, rowing, swimming. Which is best and how much is necessary to raise your fitness level steadily? If you can walk well for an hour or two, jog or run comfortably for 20 minutes, pedal at reasonable speed for 20 to 60 minutes, swim 400 to 500 strokes at your own pace, are you doing enough? And how often should you being doing this? Once a week? Twice, three times, every day?

Well, there could be an amount of exercise that is too much, a factor dependent largely on an individual's existing fitness level. Exercise is a stress but when that stress is applied carefully the body will adapt. If the levels mentioned are attained and then maintained, the fitness level will increase and that will manifest itself in shorter times to cover the same distances and in less effort being expended in the process.

The comparative oxygen and caloric costs of walking and jogging/running

Speed	Pace	Oxygen cost ml/kg/min		Caloric cost kcal/kg/min		Energy for 80kg		Energy for 60kg	
Km/h	Min/km	Walk	Jog/run	Walk	Jog/run	Kcal/min	Kcal/km	Kcal/min	Kcal/km
3.2	18.75	8.3		0.04		3.3	158	2.5	120
4.0	15.0	9.8		0.05		3.9	150	2.9	113
4.8	12.5	12.0		0.06		4.8	153	3.6	115
5.6	10.71	14.7		0.07		5.9	161	4.4	121
6.4	9.37	17.9		0.09		7.2	171	5.4	129
7.2	8.33	21.6	25.1	0.11	0.13	10.0	214	7.5	160
8.0	7.50	25.7	27.7	0.13	0.14	11.1	212	8.3	160
8.8	6.81	30.2	30.2	0.15	0.15	12.1	211	9.1	158
9.7	6.18	35.1	32.8		0.16	13.1	209	9.8	156
10.5	8.57		35.3		0.18	14.1	208	10.6	156
11.3	6.97		37.8		0.19	15.1	208	11.4	155
12.1	4.95		40.4		0.20	16.2	206	12.1	155
12.9	4.65		42.9		0.21	17.2	206	12.9	155
13.7	4.37		45.5		0.23	18.2	205	13.6	153
14.5	4.10		48.0		0.24	19.2	205	14.4	153
15.3	3.92		50.6		0.25	20.2	205	15.2	153
16.1	3.72		53.1		0.27	21.2	203	15.9	153

Extending the distances covered is then a matter of personal choice.

What happens if you take a break of a week or three weeks from your exercise programme? Not a lot unless your break happens to involve bedrest or a muscle in a cast or a flight into space. Then there can be dramatic loss of muscle tone. But carrying on normal activities, apart from the exercise routine, will see only a slight loss of fitness. One opinion is that you can, in fact, coast for months if you have established a high level of fitness but why would you want to coast at all if you are enjoying your exercise and not just the benefit it brings?

Weight-training allows you to apply resistance to specific muscles that are not challenged by regular aerobic activities so it is an important ingredient of an overall programme. It doesn't mean you have to go to a gym.

Peter once designed some exercises for the Marriott Hotel suites, which were printed in a booklet to encourage guests to work out while they were on the move. These had catchy titles such as telephone book leg-lifts, breakfast bar push-ups, bedside stomach crunches and so on.

You can make your own weights with a couple of plastic bottles, sand and a broom handle if you don't want to buy commercial weights. Arthur Lydiard once said that the best body-strengthening exercise in the world could be had from a yard of sand or gravel – you simply shovel it from one spot to another and then back again two or three times a week and work your legs, your body and your arms in unison. The important point here is to swing your shovel correctly to avoid back damage. If you have a compost heap, turn it on a regular basis. It's good for the compost as well as for you.

Recommended postures

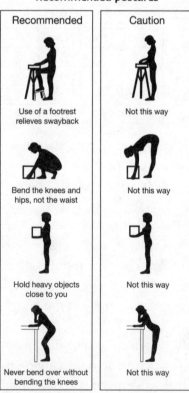

One of the great concerns of the modern lifestyle is the growing number of younger people, in their 30s or 40s, who earn enough to be able to hire housekeepers and cleaners, gardeners and lawn-care specialists and buy all the gadgets that take the effort out of household activities. They are eliminating from their lives the cheapest and most accessible sources of conditioning exercise.

There are some general principles to keep in mind, such as avoiding stress on the lower back through stooping and using the correct lifting technique by bending at the knees, which protect the lower back by keeping it straight. Examples are to the left.

The value of resistance-training

A major key to solving the problem of ageing has been the rediscovery by researchers of the value of resistance-training. The loss of muscle mass, especially as people get older, is now recognised as a primary reason for the health problems associated with ageing. While aerobic exercise, such as brisk walking or cycling, is important, it is a mistake to neglect other muscle groups not involved in either exercise.

Thus, activities involving the upper body as well as the leg muscles, such as rowing and racquet sports, are now classed as superior to walking or jogging. In fact, a study of Masters runners and cross-country skiers by Mike Pollock found that the runners lost total muscle mass with ageing, whereas the skiers, who exercise arms, legs and back muscles, maintained muscle mass. But these are not always activities that are available or attractive to many people on a basis regular enough to provide a continuing level of fitness. Walking and jogging remain the cheapest and most easily attainable forms of regular exercise.

Research has found, too, that resistance-training reduces cardio-vascular problems in the elderly. A large population study published by KR Vincent and his co-workers in a 2002 issue of the *Archives of Internal Medicine* found that, among several different exercises (weight-lifting, cycling, swimming, walking, jogging and tennis), those who performed weightlifting or jogging had the lowest incidence of coronary heart disease.

The effect of resistance-training on aerobic capacity was also investi-gated in this study. It reported that men and women aged between 60 and 83, after six months of resistance exercise three days a week for 30 minutes, improved muscle strength by between 11 and 28%, but their aerobic fitness and endurance VO_{2max} increased 23% and they were capable of exercising longer on an incremental treadmill test. This fits in with other research which suggests that the age-related decline in aerobic capacity can be explained in part by decreased muscle mass. The subjects performed 12 exercises at either low intensity or at high intensity. Progression was achieved by increasing the load by 5% when the rating of perceived exertion (RPE) dropped below 18 (see table on the following page). Results were similar for both groups in aerobic fitness, with slightly greater strength gains in the high-intensity group.

The exercises used in this study are suitable for overall strength development for all individuals:

- Leg press – quadriceps, hip extensors
- Leg curl – hamstrings
- Leg extension – quadriceps
- Overhead press – triceps
- Biceps curl – biceps
- Seated row – trapezius
- Triceps dip – triceps
- Leg abduction – abductors
- Leg adduction – adductors
- Lumbar extension – gluteals
- Abdominal crunch
- Chest press – pectorals, triceps
- Calf press – gastrocnemius, soleus

Rating of perceived exertion (RPE) and corresponding heart rates (HR) for respective age groups

RPE	Description of effort	HR 20–29	HR 30–50	HR 50–70
6	Rest	60	60	60
7	Very, very easy	70	69	67
8		80	77	74
9	Very easy	90	86	81
10	Somewhat easy	100	94	88
11	Easy	110	103	95
12		120	111	102
13	Intermediate	130	120	109
14	Somewhat hard	140	128	116
15	Hard	150	137	123
16		160	145	130
17	Very hard	170	154	137
18		180	162	144
19	Very, very hard	190	171	151
20	Exhausting – peak effort	200	179	158

Muscles that move the shoulder and arm include the trapezius and serratus anterior. The pectoralis major, latissimus dorsi, deltoid and rotator cuff muscles connect to the humerus and move the arm.

The 'why' and 'how' of resistance-training

The term 'resistance-training' once conjured up visions of sizeable men like New Zealand's Olympians Les Mills and the late Don Oliver grunting to lift barbells of enormous weight. Not any more.

Today, men, women and children of all ages pursue and benefit from resistance-training. When you apply resistance to a muscle or muscle groups, the muscle fibres are activated to work against that resistance and receive a stimulus to increase the amount of contractile protein they contain, which ultimately increases strength – hence the use of both terms.

In addition to the increase in muscle protein, there is a neural component, in which the ability to activate a larger fraction of the muscle is enhanced, resulting in an apparent rapid increase in strength. You need sufficient strength for activities such as golf, cycling, tennis, skiing and dancing just as much as you do for physically demanding occupational tasks, such as construction and firefighting.

Possession of adequate strength can save your life – not only by allowing you to repel an attacker but by enabling you to escape from a crisis situation, such as a burning building. Strength can also save the lives of the elderly by preventing falls.

Resistance-training is especially important as we reach our 50s when arthritic pain and a possible decline in the secretion of natural hormones, such as growth hormone (GH) and testosterone, act to reduce activity levels and lead, ultimately, to a loss of strength.

In addition to fitness activities, anyone who grocery shops, runs after children or works around the house needs strength. Seems like everyone is included.

Resistance-training is simply finding a way to increase the load on a muscle or muscle group. Arthur Lydiard did not advocate the use of weights for his runners but instead had them use the *resistance of gravity* by running up hills to increase leg strength.

Selecting the correct weight

Heavy weights should be avoided in the beginning. Excessive weight will contribute little to strength development and only serves to increase the chance of injury. Using a lighter resistance and more repetitions (reps) is advised when beginning a weight-training programme. A novice should be able to complete 12 to 15 reps. So, how do you go about choosing an appropriate weight? As an example, consider a typical health club bench-press exercise as shown below.

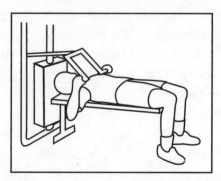

Pick the lightest weight on the stack (usually 4.5kg) and see how it feels to lift this weight a few times. Add a little more weight and see how that feels, again for three or four repetitions. Repeat this process until you find a weight you can lift eight to10 times without straining too hard – maybe 18kg to 27kg. This is your starting weight. The goal will be to increase this weight over time as strength improves. Generally, if you can do 12 repetitions of an exercise without a huge effort, you should consider adding 2.25kg to 4.5kg. With this extra weight, you may be limited to eight repetitions. This is okay because your goal will be to accomplish 12 repetitions before moving on. This process is used for all exercises, the weight or resistance varying according to your ability to do the movement.

Understanding the movements

When using weights to increase muscular strength, the movement is called dynamic, because there is a change in muscle length. There are two types of dynamic activity: concentric and eccentric. Concentric activity occurs when the muscle shortens, as in a biceps curl, moving the weight from a low position to a high one. Eccentric action occurs when the weight is lowered and the muscle lengthens. The eccentric action is very important and should be done slowly and purposefully.

Running downhill involves eccentric muscle contraction and is used in the laboratory on a down-sloping treadmill to study the effects of muscle soreness arising from microscopic tears in the eccentrically contracting muscles.

Both eccentric and concentric activity are important to ensure muscle/strength balance. Most exercises have an eccentric component but most people have been in the habit of not appreciating its value and just letting the weights flop. For example, when doing a push-up, the body should be lowered from full-arm extension in a controlled manner, not in a collapse.

Muscles to work on

Runners, walkers and cyclists use the large muscles in the legs. These are the quadriceps, the large muscle in the front of the leg, and the hamstrings, the opposing muscle in the back of the leg, and they provide the ability to lift the leg. To strengthen the 'quads', the best movements are squats and knee extensions. You don't even need weights. Work up to 20 reps with feet together and 20 reps with feet apart and pointing out.

The angle at the knee joint affects the leverage and the stress placed on the joint so be careful about bending the knee too much – especially older knees like ours. A half or quarter squat will be beneficial whereas a full squat might wreck those ageing knees. If using resistance, do leg presses. A leg press is like a squat but is done on a machine in the sitting position with the back supported. To strengthen hamstrings, do hamstring curls. Stand straight and lift the heel to the buttock. Doing calf raises can strengthen calves.

Raising onto the toes with a barbell on the shoulders is an excellent exercise for not only the large calf muscles but all those around the ankle that are used in walking, running, hopping, jumping and skipping. The muscles (gastrocnemius, soleus, peroneus longus and brevis, flexor hallucis longus, tibialis posterior and flexor digitorum longus) are all involved in plantar flexion of the foot and contribute to ankle strength and stability. (Aren't you glad you asked?) Flexibility is enhanced when joints are moved through a full range of motion.

Strengthening the upper body helps to maintain good running form and will assist in reducing overall fatigue. To strengthen biceps, do biceps curls, focusing on the eccentric action, or pull-ups on a horizontal bar (chins) with the palms of the hands facing towards you as you grip the bar. To achieve strong shoulders, do upright rows and lateral arm raises. In upright rowing, a barbell (or bar connected to pulley weights) is held in front of the body with the hands close together and the arms extended. The bar is then lifted to the top of the chest in a motion that is not unlike rowing. Lateral arm raises are simply extending the arms from the side of the body to the horizontal position. They are good for the many muscles around the shoulder joint – the so-called rotator cuff.

One of Peter's favourites (no weights needed) is the push-up. These work the arms, chest and back. Modified push-ups, with our knees on the floor, are a good way to achieve 20-plus reps, which many people would find impossible at the start. This goes for men, too.

One of the most important muscle groups to strengthen is the abdominals. The trunk area is known as the 'core' and a strong core helps you to maintain form, reduce back injuries and aches, and also helps you to breathe better. Sit-ups can assist you to achieve that strong core. Crunches, with knees bent and hands behind your head for support, are recommended. While lifting straight up, getting the shoulder blades off the floor, you work the rectus abdominis, the big muscle down the centre of the abdomen. Moving the shoulder towards the opposite knee works the obliques, the muscles on each side. But a word of caution: the full sit-up, which is raising head and shoulders up to the knees, may aggravate back pain. If you are at risk of lower back pain you should avoid it. Starting with your back flat on the floor can lead to a jerky movement. Lowering from a position about 15cm off the floor is more controlled.

A recent research finding is that one set of exercises is as effective as multiple sets. This indicates that the most important factor for the development of strength is the quality or intensity of the exercise and not the quantity or volume. The intensity of the exercise defines how many muscle fibres are activated to overcome the resistance and perform the movement. Remember that, in general, a muscle fibre must contract for a training adaptation to occur so it follows that the more fibres are contracted the better.

Repetition recommendations

Healthy sedentary adults	Sets; RM	No of exercises*	Frequency
1998 ACSM Position Stand	1 set; 8–12 RM	8–10	2–3 days/week
1998 ACSM Guidelines	1 set; 8–12 RM	8–10	2 days/week minimum
1996 Surgeon General's Report	1–2 set; 8–12 RM	8–10	2 days/week
Elderly persons			
Pollock et al (1994)	1 set; 10–15 RM	8–10	2 days/week minimum
Cardiac patients			
1995 AHA Exercise Standards	1 set; 10–15 RM	8–10	2–3 days/week
1995 AACVPR Guidelines	1 set; 10–15 RM	8–10	2–3 days/week

* Minimum one exercise per major muscle group.

Abbreviations: ACSM: American College of Sports Medicine; AHA: American Heart Association; AACVPR: American Association of Cardiovascular & Pulmonary Rehabilitation.

Note: These recommendations refer to the repetition max method (e.g., the most weight that can be lifted for 8-12 repetitions). However, this is for optimal results and it is always prudent to start off slowly and progress, with equal patience, to higher resistance/loads.

Exercises for major muscle groups

Muscle groups	Specific muscles	Exercises
Shoulders, arms, upper back	Deltoids, trapezius, biceps, triceps, latissimus dorsi, erector spinae	Bicep curls, 'rowing' exercise, push-ups, chinning the bar
Midsection or core	Abdominals, obliques, lower back	Abdominal & oblique sit-ups & crunches, lower back extensions
Hip	Hip flexors (ilio-psoas), hip extensors (gluteals, hamstrings)	Straight single-leg lifts from a supine position and the same exercise in a prone position
Lower body – thigh, calf, ankle and foot	Leg adductors and abductors, quadriceps, hamstrings, calf muscles, ankle extensors – plantar flexion, gastrocnemius	Knee extensions, squats, knee flexion (curls), toe raises

From these research findings, the recommendations as shown in the table on the previous page have changed from three sets to one set. The term RM stands for repetition maximum and is qualified by a number, for example 1RM is the maximum amount of weight that can be lifted in a single effort; eight to 10 RM means the maximum amount of weight that can be lifted for eight to 10 times for each exercise.

Some muscles span two joints and can be exercised with more than one type of movement. For example, the major muscle of the calf, the gastrocnemius, attaches to the Achilles tendon and is primarily used in lifting the heel (toe raises) when the knee is straight (the soleus is more active when the knee is bent and the gastrocnemius shortened). However, because the gastrocnemius originates above the knee joint, it is also activated to assist the hamstrings in knee flexion. Likewise, the main hamstrings muscle (rectus femoris), which originates above the hip joint, not only flexes the knee, but also pulls the leg back (hip extension). Thus, it is possible to be creative in deciding on a programme of resistance exercises.

Basic tips for resistance-training

Do warm-ups, such as marching in place or jumping jacks. Before heading out on a run after age 40, Peter learnt that he could avoid calf muscle strains by doing a minute of heel raises.

Resistance-train at least twice a week to notice benefits. You can work all the muscles mentioned above in 20 minutes. Training, especially high-intensity training, involves a process of damage and repair. The 'damage' is not obvious, but involves tiny tears in connective tissue that recuperate rapidly, unlike a strain or gross tear that you can feel and pinpoint. It should not be thought of as a negative but as a stimulus causing favourable adaptation. However, we need to allow adequate time for recovery, which is why successive days of heavy resistance-training should be avoided.

If it hurts, don't do it.

Increased muscle mass helps burn fat and calories.

Building muscle mass increases bone density. This can help to maintain strong bones as we age. This goes for both men and women and particularly Third Agers.

Don't forget to breathe properly during resistance workouts. Straining while holding your breath causes blood pressure to rise markedly. Therefore, it is recommended that you always exhale during the effort phase. It is believed that the sudden exhalation of air aids muscular activity. Listen to the grunts, shouts and groans of weightlifters, shot-putters and tennis players. These days, even golfers are grunting at the moment of impact.

When just beginning a weight-training programme, involving free weights and machines, it is advisable to work with, or at the least consult, a fitness trainer, study instructional videos or seek out a very knowledgeable friend willing to help you on your way down the right road.

Remember that building a strong body not only assists you in running and other fitness activities, but it also reduces the risk of coronary heart disease, lowers blood pressure in some people and helps you to deal more effectively with the daily demands of work and play.

CHAPTER NINE

The Effects of Exercise

Specific effects of exercise

As we have explained in considerable but necessary detail, sensible regular exercise can add healthy and active years to your life. Moderately fit people, even if they smoke or have high blood pressure, have a lower mortality rate than the least fit. Studies continue to show that it is never too late to start exercising and even those small improvements in physical fitness and activity at any age can significantly lower the risk of death. Simply walking regularly can prolong life and independent living in the elderly. Even in nursing homes, patients on programmes aimed at improving strength, balance, gait and flexibility gain significant benefits. So let's take a detailed look at how exercise affects the ills and ailments, aches and pains of advancing years. If you find some of this material repetitive, we make no apologies. Every repetition is a reminder to you of the need to look after yourself thoughtfully and carefully, not to add years to your life – although this could happen – but to make the years you have more enjoyable. And repetition is a vital element of whatever exercise regime you choose to follow

Resistance-training is particularly important for the elderly because it is the only form of exercise that can slow and even reverse the decline in muscle mass, bone density and strength. As little as one day a week of resistance-training improves overall strength and agility – but two to three days is even better.

Adding workouts that involve fast movements may be even more protective for older people. For example, slow continuous jogging is good aerobic exercise, but a short period (one to two minutes) of faster running, followed by a one-minute walk, activates more muscle mass. Of course, do not push yourself so hard that one minute is not sufficient time to recover. Flexibility exercises promote healthy muscle growth and help reduce the stiffness and loss of balance that accompanies ageing, easing those activities.

Cardiovascular health

Inactivity is one of the four major risk factors for heart disease, on a par with smoking, unhealthy cholesterol and even high blood pressure. Like all muscles, the heart becomes stronger and larger as a result of exercise so it can pump more blood through the body with every beat. Exercise does not increase the maximum heart rate but *a fit heart can pump more blood at this maximum level and can sustain it longer with less strain.* The resting heart rate of those who exercise is also slower because less effort is needed to pump blood. For preventing heart disease, frequency of exercises may be more important than duration. Exercise helps improve heart health in people with many forms of heart disease and can even reverse some risk factors, such as the effects of smoking. Unfortunately, studies show that those with the highest heart risks (such as smokers and people who are overweight) and who would most benefit from exercise are the least likely to persist.

Coronary artery disease and cholesterol levels

People who maintain an active lifestyle have a 45% lower risk of developing coronary heart disease than do sedentary people. Studies report that people who change their diet in order to control cholesterol and lower the risk of coronary artery disease are successful only when they also follow a regular aerobic exercise programme. Brisk walking, jogging, swimming, biking, aerobic dance and racquet sports are the best forms of exercise for reducing blood triglyceride levels (harmful fat molecules which can be stored in the wrong places such as the liver) and raising HDL ('good' cholesterol) levels. It may take up to a year of sustained exercise for HDL levels to show significant improvement.

Aerobic exercise also appears to open up the blood vessels and, in combination with a healthy diet, may improve blood–clotting factors.

Burning at least 300 calories a day (the equivalent of about 45 minutes of brisk walking or 25 minutes of jogging) seems to confer the greatest protection against coronary artery disease. Even moderate exercise, however, reduces the risk of heart attack but, in terms of raising HDL levels, more is better. Resistance-training offers a complementary benefit by reducing LDL ('bad' cholesterol) levels. Triglycerides, which rise after a high-fat meal, can be lowered either with a single, prolonged (about 90 minutes) aerobic session or by several shorter sessions during the day.

High blood pressure

Studies indicate that regular exercise helps keep arteries elastic, even in older people, which in turn improves blood flow and blood pressure. Sedentary people have a 35% greater risk of developing hypertension than athletes do. No person with high blood pressure should start an exercise programme without consulting a doctor.

Studies have shown that high-intensity exercise may not lower blood pressure as effectively as moderate intensity exercise. In one study, for example, moderate exercise (jogging 3km a day) controlled hypertension so well that more than half the patients who had been taking drugs for high blood pressure were able to discontinue their medication.

Other studies have indicated that t'ai chi may lower blood pressure almost as well as moderate-intensity aerobic exercises. Before exercising, people with hypertension should avoid caffeinated drinks, which increase heart rate, the workload of the heart and blood pressure during physical activity.

Stroke

The benefits of exercise on stroke are uncertain. According to an analysis of a group of 11,000 men, followed for 12 years in the Harvard Alumni Study, those who burned between 2000 and 3000 calories a week (about an hour of brisk walking five days a week) cut their risk of stroke in half. Groups who burned between 1000 and 2000 calories or more than 3000 calories a week also gained some protection against stroke but to a lesser degree. In the same study, exercise that involved recreation was more protective than exercise routines consisting simply of walking or climbing.

Heart failure

Traditionally, heart failure patients have been discouraged from exercising. Now exercise performed under medical supervision is proving to be helpful for selected patients with stable heart failure. In one study, patients between the ages of 61 and 91 increased their oxygen consumption by 20% after six months by engaging in supervised treadmill and stationary bicycle exercises.

In New Zealand the Lydiard principle of jogging actually had its origins with recovering heart attack patients. It has since been shown to have been very effective in bringing some heart patients back to such a stage of fitness that they have run – at their own pace – full 42km marathons.

Diabetes

Diabetes, particularly type 2, is reaching epidemic proportions throughout the world as more and more cultures adopt bad Western dietary habits and sedentary lifestyles. But regular aerobic exercise is proving to have significant benefits for people with type 2 diabetes; it increases sensitivity to insulin, lowers blood pressure, improves cholesterol level, and decreases body fat. Studies of older people who engage in regular, moderate aerobic exercise (e.g., brisk walking and biking) indicates they lower their risk for diabetes even if they don't lose weight. Anyone on insulin or who has complications from diabetes must take special precautions before embarking on a workout programme.

Bones and joints

Osteoarthritis

Exercise helps to reduce pain and stiffness and increases flexibility, muscle strength, endurance and well-being. Osteoarthritis patients should avoid high-impact sports, such as jogging, tennis and squash. The three types of exercise that are best for people with arthritis are range of motion, resistance and aerobic exercises. Strengthening exercises include isometric exercises (pushing or pulling against static resistance) and stretching exercises to build strength and flexibility without unduly stressing the joints. These exercises may be particularly important if leg muscle weakness turns out to be a cause of osteoarthritis, as some research suggests.

Low-impact aerobics also help to stabilise and support the joints and may even reduce inflammation in some joints. Cycling and walking are beneficial, and swimming or exercising in water is highly recommended for people with arthritis or while recovering from leg injury.

One study compared a group of patients who embarked on an aerobic and resistance exercise programme with a group that received patient education; the exercising group developed less disability and pain and showed a better ability to perform physical tasks.

Patients should strive for short but frequent exercise sessions guided by physical therapists or certified instructors.

Osteoporosis

Exercise is very important for slowing the progression of osteoporosis. Women should begin exercising before adolescence since bone mass increases during puberty and reaches its peak between ages 20 and 30. Weight-bearing exercise, which applies tension to muscle and bone, encourages the body to compensate for the added stress by increasing bone density by as much as 2% to 8% a year. High-impact weight-bearing exercises, such as step aerobics, protect bone density from deteriorating in women. These exercises, however, increase the risk of osteoporotic fractures in elderly patients, who would benefit most from regular, brisk, long walks.

Even moderate exercise (as little as an hour a week) helps reduce the risk of fracture, but everyone who is in good health should aim for more. Careful weight-training is beneficial as well for older women. Low-impact exercises that improve balance and strength, particularly yoga and t'ai chi, have been found to decrease the risk of falling; in one study, t'ai chi reduced the risk by almost half.

Back problems

One of the most common complaints of modern men and women, lower-back pain afflicts up to 80% of all Americans. Sedentary living, obesity, poor posture, badly designed furniture and stress all contribute to back pain. An appropriate exercise programme focusing on flexibility and strengthening the muscles in the abdomen may help prevent back problems. Yoga stretching is beneficial and can be incorporated into the warm-up and cool-down periods.

The best exercises for people with bad backs include swimming and walking. High-impact sports, including aerobic dance and downhill skiing, should be avoided. Exercises that strengthen the abdominal muscles, such as partial sit-ups, which maintain the back's normal curve and help support the body's weight, can alleviate stress on the lower back. However, the classic full sit-up (raising your head and shoulders off the floor up to your knees) may aggravate back pain and should be avoided by anyone at risk of lower-back problems.

About 20% of weight-training injuries involve the lower back. Improper exercise instruction and inattention to the proper use of equipment can be sources of trouble. A single jerky golf swing or incorrect use of exercise equipment, especially free weights, rowing machines and the huge range of home-gym equipment can cause serious back injuries. One small study on competitive rowers suggests that for people who use rowing machines, breathing out during the drive segment of the stroke may offer some protection for the lower back.

Lung disease

Although exercise does not improve lung function per se, training helps many patients with chronic obstructive lung disease (COPD) by strengthening their limb muscles, thus improving endurance and reducing breathlessness.

Cancer

A number of studies have indicated that regular, even moderate, exercise reduces the risk of colon cancer and, in fact, any cancer related to obesity. Moderate exercise has been shown to reduce the risk of breast cancer and strenuous activity may lower the risk of prostate cancer.

A long-term study of 100,000 nurses, however, suggested that the benefits of exercise on breast health may be greater or lesser at different times in a woman's life, depending on her menstrual status and oestrogen levels. For example, the study found no added protection from exercise in young adulthood (when the disease is uncommon in any case).

Several studies are under way to measure the effect of exercise on patients who have been diagnosed with cancer. Even though preliminary, they already suggest that exercise has a positive physical, mental and emotional effect. Exercise can improve physical strength, functional capacity and the ability to battle the negative side-effects of chemotherapy, including nausea and fatigue. More studies are warranted.

Infectious illness

The effect of exercise on the immune system varies with intensity and regularity. Although offering no evidence of improved immunity from exercise, one study reported that people who exercised as little as once a week in employee fitness programmes averaged nearly five fewer sick days annually than those who did not participate in such programmes. Other studies have also indicated that regular vigorous exercise improves immune function. In people who already have colds, exercise has no effect on the illness's severity or the duration of the infection.

People should avoid strenuous physical activity when they have high fevers or widespread viral illnesses, however. High-intensity or endurance exercises appear to suppress the immune system while they are being performed. Some highly trained athletes, for instance, report being susceptible to colds after strenuous events and during periods of hard training. Very low-fat diets appear to support this negative effect on the immune system. A higher-fat diet may help redress this imbalance (omega-3 fatty acids, found in cold-water fish, canola oil and flaxseed oil, are preferred). Whether carbohydrate loading provides much additional value is not clear.

Central nervous system diseases

People with multiple sclerosis, Parkinson's disease and Alzheimer's disease should be encouraged to exercise. Specialised exercise programmes that improve mobility are particularly valuable for Parkinson's patients. Patients with neurological disorders who exercise experience less spasticity as well as reduction in, and even reversal of, muscle atrophy.

In addition, the psychological benefits of exercise are extremely important in managing these disorders. Exercise machines, aquatic exercises and walking are particularly useful.

Pregnancy

Healthy women with normal pregnancies should exercise at least three times a week, being careful to warm up, cool down and drink plenty of liquids. Many prenatal callisthenics programmes are available. Experts advise, in general, that when exercising, the expectant mother's pulse rate should not exceed 70 to 75% of the maximum heart rate or more than 150 beats/minute. In one study previously sedentary low-risk pregnant women exercised to 150 to 156 beats/minute three times a week without any harmful effects, but any woman who did not exercise intensely before becoming pregnant should check with her doctor before embarking on such a programme.

Fit women who have exercised regularly before pregnancy may work out intensely as long as no discomfort occurs. According to one study, vigorous exercise may improve the chances of a timely delivery. All pregnant women should avoid high-impact, jerky and jarring exercises, such as aerobic dancing, which can weaken the pelvic floor muscles that support the uterus. During exercise, women should monitor their temperature to avoid overheating, a side-effect that can damage the foetus. No pregnant women should use hot tubs or steam baths, which can cause foetal damage and miscarriage.

Swimming and water aerobics may be the best option for most pregnant women and have special benefits for those with fluid retention. Water exercises involve no impact, overheating is unlikely and swimming face down promotes optimum blood flow to the uterus. Performing yoga exercises under the guidance of informed instructors can be very helpful. Walking is highly beneficial. And to strengthen pelvic muscles, women should perform Kegel exercises at least six times a day, which involve contracting the muscles around the vagina and urethra for three seconds 12 to 15 times in a row.

An American College of Obstetrics and Gynecology study suggests that most pregnant women in the US are not getting enough exercise. Ideally, if they do not have any medical or obstetric complications, they should participate in at least 30 minutes of moderate physical activity on most days of the week, the same level recommended for everyone.

'There appears to be a discrepancy between the professional recommendations for physical activity during pregnancy and what women have actually been doing,' said Dr Ann Petersen and colleagues at Saint Louis University in St Louis, Missouri, as reported in *Medicine & Science in Sports & Exercise.*

The findings suggest that 'the message regarding physical activity during pregnancy is not being heard or is not being perceived as important by most pregnant women, although research shows that pregnant women who are physically active are less likely to gain excessive weight during their pregnancy and less likely to develop complications, [such as] gestational diabetes and pregnancy-induced hypertension', co-author Dr Terry Leet told Reuters Health.

Few studies have investigated the frequency, duration and type of activity that women perform while pregnant, and those that have did not focus on whether the women met the recommended guidelines.

To investigate, the college researchers analysed data collected by telephone in 1994, 1996, 1998 and 2000 from more than 150,000 women, 6528 of whom were pregnant. All the women were between the ages of 18 and 44.

Dr Leet said only one of every six pregnant women compared to one of every four non-pregnant women was meeting the recommended guidelines.

In 1994, for example, 28% of non-pregnant women reported participating in regular vigorous or moderate physical activity, compared with 20% of pregnant women. In 2000, 27% of non-pregnant women met the guidelines for moderate physical activity, compared with just 16% of pregnant women.

Walking was the most common activity among the women, reported by 52% of pregnant women and 45% of non-pregnant women. Fewer pregnant women than non-pregnant women reported participating in aerobics, running/jogging, gardening or swimming laps.

For each year included in the analysis, however, at least 33% of pregnant women reported not participating in any physical activity. Among non-pregnant women, about 25% reported participating in no physical activity each year.

Injuries from high-impact exercise

About half the people at any age who participate in competitive running or high-impact aerobics experience minor injuries at least once a year. Young, intensely competitive athletes may be at risk for permanent injury. Studies are conflicting over whether intensive high-impact sports in younger people cause long-term degenerative joint disease.

Older people should embark on vigorous activity with caution. Between 1990 and 1996, injuries from active sports increased by 54% in people aged 65 and older. Women are far more likely than men to rupture a knee ligament, although a combination of weightlifting and jumping exercises may prevent injury by strengthening hamstrings and improving coordination.

Urinary incontinence affects many women who engage in high-impact exercise. Shock-absorbing footwear and weight-dampening inserts may help prevent this problem.

High-impact exercise can also damage the inner ear, causing dizziness, ringing in the ear, motion sickness, or loss of high-frequency hearing. To avoid injuries, you should vary your training and alternate easy and harder workouts. You should also be careful to warm up, cool down, and stretch; flexibility is the key to preventing many muscle strains. You should also take days off now and then; the risk of injury increases when you train more than five times a week.

Treating minor injuries

Most mild or moderate injuries respond well to a simple, four-step treatment: rest, ice, compression and elevation (RICE). This regime works well for both acute injuries and chronic problems. Ice packs, which minimise inflammation and pain, can help acute injuries and can be useful for the first few hours after a chronically injured area is exercised. Heat, ultrasound, whirlpool and massage may speed healing if applied a day or two after the initial injury or for the warm-up before another workout session.

Water wisdom

Perhaps this is a good point at which to mention the value of water, often called the neglected nutrient. And to remind you that at the moment you feel thirsty you are already mildly dehydrated.

Water regulates body temperature, removes body waste, carries nutrients, oxygen and glucose to the cells to give you energy, naturally moistens the skin and other tissues, cushions joints and helps strengthen muscles, keeps stools softer and maximises mental function.

Inadequate water intake can slow thinking ability, cause forgetfulness, headaches, loss of balance, constipation, diverticular disease and kidney stones, impair blood flow and give you dry skin, eyes and mouth.

As you age, the dehydration risk increases because older people have less sensitivity to thirst, have a fear of incontinence, have trouble swallowing, may have difficulty in holding a cup or glass and have decreased kidney function.

You need to drink 31ml of water a day for every kilogram of bodyweight. A 68kg person thus needs 2108ml to be adequately hydrated.

The colour of your urine is an excellent indicator: clear to pale yellow denotes adequate hydration; dark yellow to gold means you need to drink more water. Urinating at least every two hours is another indication that you are drinking enough water.

Drink water in slow sips. Gulping it down can cause gastric distress.

If you don't drink enough water, your kidneys must compensate by excreting more concentrated urine, which may lead to the formation of kidney stones – a very painful condition when they pass through the urethra.

During exercise lasting less than 60 minutes, water is the preferred drink. Electrolyte replacement is not necessary and the sugar in sports drinks provides empty calories. If you lose 0.5kg during an exercise session, drink at least half a litre of water.

Calculate your needs from this table:

Your water needs

Weight (kg)	Litres/day
18–22.5	1.5
23–27	1.6
27.5–31.5	1.7
32–36	1.7
36.5–44.5	1.8
45–54	1.5 to 1.8
54.5–63	1.8 to 2
63.5–72	2 to 2.4
72.5–84	2 to 2.6
85+	3

A table to keep track of your daily and weekly intake is suggested as a way of making sure you meet your water needs. Like any training schedule, it's a good disciplinarian. Something like on the following page, for example:

Water intake

	Typical	Monday	Tuesday	Wednesday	Thursday	Friday	Saturday	Sunday
Wake up								
Breakfast								
Mid-morning								
Lunch								
Mid-afternoon								
Dinner								
Evening								
Before bed								

And a warning

The body is capable of excreting a large amount of water, but in some cases, usually among non-elite marathon runners, too much water intake will dilute the plasma sodium and cause hyponatraemia, a potentially dangerous condition. The fluid balance across the blood-brain barrier becomes disrupted, resulting in a rapid influx of water into the brain. This causes brain swelling and a cascade of increasingly severe neurological responses (headache, malaise, confusion, seizure, coma) that can lead to death. The body normally regulates sodium levels by excreting excess through sweating and the kidneys.

Dehydration

Everyone should drink lots of fluid during intense exercise. Thirst is often a poor indicator of dehydration in people who exercise, particularly older people, and they often underestimate the amount of fluid they need. During a tough workout in a hot environment, the body can lose two litres of fluid per hour through sweat. Athletes should drink 175 to 230 millilitres of fluid about 15 minutes before a workout, and then pause regularly during exercise for more.

Contrary to popular belief, drinking fluids will not cause cramps. Adequate hydration, in fact, helps prevent the painful involuntary muscle spasms that sometimes occur during exercise. Water is effective for replenishing body fluids. However, during prolonged exercise in the heat, 'sports drinks' that contain glucose, sodium and potassium are more effective than water at improving endurance. Caffeinated drinks like coffee and soft drinks give short bursts of energy but can actually reduce body fluid through their diuretic effect.

According to one study, caffeine before a workout temporarily raises blood pressure and reduces blood flow to inactive limbs, suggesting that those with hypertension and possibly anyone who exercises in hot weather should avoid it. This action of caffeine is due to the constriction of blood vessels, an effect which is overridden by the dilating stimulus of exercise in contracting muscles.

The signs of dehydration

% loss of body water	Signs of dehydration
0 to 1%	Thirst
2 to 5%	Dry mouth, flushed skin, fatigue, headache, impaired physical performance
6%	Increased body temperature, breathing rate and pulse rate
8%	Dizziness, increased weakness, difficulty breathing with exertion
10%	Muscle spasms, swollen tongue, delirium
11%	Poor blood circulation, failing kidney function

Sweat those germs away

An entire industry has been built around the need to disguise the fact that people sweat. Sweat is something we almost inevitably produce in abundance when we exercise and commonly produce even when we don't, but it has become one of the social stigmas of our time, and pharmaceutical companies enjoy handsome profits from deodorants and antiperspirants.

Now the findings of a German study suggest sweat could be a lifesaver because it contains a germ-fighting agent that may work against infection. Dr Birgit Schittek and colleagues at Eberhard-Karls University in Tübingen isolated the gene responsible for the compound. According to the journal *Nature Immunology*, they have called the gene, and the protein it produces, dermicidin. Schittek believes dermicidin could possibly limit an infection very early, which makes sweating a first line of defence.

The agent is manufactured in the sweat glands, secreted in the sweat and taken to the skin's surface. Dr Schittek says dermicidin is the first antimicrobial found that is produced by cells in the human skin and is consistently produced to provide a constant protection against invading micro-organisms. They found it was active against many different types of bacteria, including normal inhabitants of the intestines, which can infect wounds or cause contamination.

Maybe, in time, sweat will become an accepted health statement and, instead of running off to the pharmacy for something to clean up an infection, you can go for a run.

So, all is not lost in sweat; nor is all lost to the natural processes of ageing. Plenty of proof exists that ageing can be countered by virtually anyone.

Hyperthermia

Overheating, or hyperthermia, is closely related to dehydration and can be a problem with strenuous exercise or when working out in hot weather. Overheating can cause mild to life-threatening conditions. Heat exhaustion, a moderate form of hyperthermia, is characterised by light-headedness, nausea, headache, hyperventilation, fatigue and loss of concentration. Although the victim's temperature will be high (above 43°C), he or she may complain of chills and the skin may be clammy.

Individuals should rest in a cool, dry place, drink plenty of fluids and bring down their body temperature with ice packs pressed against the skin.

Heatstroke is the most dangerous complication of hyperthermia. The victim may suddenly cease sweating, after which symptoms such as altered consciousness, seizures, and even coma may quickly follow. Heatstroke is a medical emergency and requires immediate cooling of the victim in an ice-water bath or with ice packs. One study suggests that the risk of serious complications from exercising in high temperatures may persist as late as the following day, even if the weather has cooled down.

Frostbite and hypothermia

Precautions also need to be taken in cold weather. When exercising in winter, dress in layers, including gloves and socks, which create insulated air pockets that trap heat. In cold weather, wear shoes with less ventilation than those worn in the summer. Fingers, toes, ears and nose are most susceptible to frostbite. From stinging or aching, frostbite progresses to numbness. Fingers and toes may become white. Soaking the extremities in warm water can help, but only once there is no risk of refreezing, since a second bout of frostbite after thawing can accelerate tissue damage.

Hypothermia can be life-threatening and can occur even in temperatures that are above freezing after prolonged exposure. The condition is characterised by extreme fatigue, mental confusion, apathy and a lack of coordination. The victim should be warmed as soon as possible with blankets, body heat and warm fluids.

Medications

If medications of any kind are part of your life, you should consult your doctor to make sure that exercising is safe. For example, the use of anabolic steroids to stimulate the production of muscle tissue is unfortunately on the rise; it is very dangerous and can increase the risk of stroke and heart attack. The group of cholesterol-lowering drugs known as statins and taken by millions has been associated with muscle disease in a small number of patients.

It is recommended that individuals with unexplained muscle pain or weakness who are taking statins should see their doctor and that intense exercise should be avoided until the cause of the muscle symptoms is determined. Some antihypertensive drugs such as diuretics and betablockers, the latter attenuating heart rate and force of ventricular contraction, tend to reduce athletic performance but should not be a reason to refrain from regular exercise.

CHAPTER TEN

Your Time Is Now All Yours

Fulfilment and activities – life after family

Well, your family has grown up, their education is complete and they have gone to begin new lives away from the nest. The other demands of establishing security and a sound upbringing for them are also gone. Your own future security has been taken care of. Retirement is approaching – or may even have arrived.

Now what are you going to do with the sudden arrival of a new kind of freedom?

This is a challenge that needs careful thinking. You can seize the chance to expand your horizons, bring from the corners of your mind those ambitions that have been lurking there but never seemed achievable, or change the directions of your interests and your life entirely if you want to.

Peter has always taken the position that, while your body is capable, you should do the strenuous activities – racquet sports, basketball, hockey, triathlons, skiing, soccer, backpacking, mountaineering, trail biking, orienteering, white-water rafting, sailing and so on. The less strenuous activities can follow – perhaps golf, bowls, fishing, boating, tramping or cycling.

Peter loves golf and he believes he will get as much pleasure playing when he is 70 as he did in his 20s when he played to a 12 handicap in New Zealand. The only caveat to this advice is that the skills are easier to acquire at a younger age but, once learnt, the movements remain in the muscle memory and can be recalled in a relatively short time.

Peter has some items still on his list of things to do in New Zealand:

- Walk the Milford Track.
- Ski down the Tasman Glacier.
- Canoe the length of the Whanganui River from Taumarunui to Pipiriki – skipping the boring part from Pipiriki down to the coast.

It is critical to have a wide variety of interests to keep the mind alert, the imagination alive and the motivation there to make every day a day to look forward to.

Garth has his eyes on the annual 169km cycle event round Lake Taupo. Despite serious undertraining, he tackled it two years ago but was forced to quit after 100km of a succession of steep hills into a mounting headwind. He still undertrains, simply for lack of time between writing and other requirements of a busy life. He is also hanging on to his mid-teens golf handicap and, who knows, if he lives long enough, looks forward to playing a round that equals his age. His positive view is that it becomes more achievable every year – right now, he can only go eight over his course par of 71 but, when he's 100, he can play 29 over.

Even if he doesn't make it, he is enjoying the challenge of trying to rebuild a golf swing and mental approach that equate to his age now but may give him the results he enjoyed when he was much younger. His rationale: you never know until you try and if you don't try you'll never know.

Orienteering is Peter's favourite activity at present. It is a sport which can have a strong competitive element but can just as easily be done for personal accomplishment and the enjoyment of the outdoors. Orienteering has the advantage of being more than a foot race; it is also a mental challenge because you use a detailed colour map and compass to find, in a specific order, a series of points located on features marked on the map and revealed on the ground with coloured flags. The route to be followed to reach each marker in turn as quickly as possible is part of the decision-making required. The level of fitness is not as important as in, say, cross-country racing or half-marathons, which many Third Agers are drawn to as the fitness bug bites. When Peter was in his late 20s, he went out to the Woodhill Forest near Auckland with Ralph King and Gordon Pirie to 'try orienteering'. It didn't appeal at the time, probably because he was still interested in purely physical contests and the navigation component made him look mediocre. He was reminded of this when watching the Eco Challenge race in Fiji in 2003 in which many good competitors saw their hopes dashed by mistakes in navigation.

Quick reminders for staying healthy

As the medical profession broadens its interest in and knowledge of longevity, the more it becomes evident that lifestyle plays a significant role in how long and how well people live. It is probable that lifestyle is more than twice as important as genes in getting you into the Third Age in good shape and condition, physically and mentally.

That being so, let's run through those lifestyle aspects that you can control to improve the odds in your favour.

Monitor your cholesterol

Heart disease leads the race as the killer of both men and women, so have a cholesterol test, especially if you haven't even thought about it for the past five years or so. Ideally, your total cholesterol level should be less than 5.17 mmol/1. Your HDL should be 1.03 mmol/1 or higher; your LDL should be less than 3.35 mmol/1. In some cases the total cholesterol may be high due to high levels of HDL, therefore a ratio of total cholesterol to HDL is a more accurate indicator.

For example, person A with the recommended values of 5.17 mmol/1 and 1.03 mmol/1 has a ratio of 5.0, whereas person B with 'moderately high' cholesterol of 5.69 mmol/1 and an HDL of 1.29 mmol/1 has a much better ratio of 4.4. Generally, a ratio of less than five is desirable, but again the lower the better.

The reason for this apparent paradox is that the total cholesterol is comprised of the LDL and HDL fractions and also a small amount packaged with circulating triglycerides or VLDL. With normal to moderately high triglycerides the cholesterol component is estimated as 1/5 of the triglyceride concentration. To summarise:

Total cholesterol = LDL cholesterol + HDL cholesterol + 1/5 VLDL

Low-density lipoprotein is the major cholesterol carrier in the blood and, as discussed earlier, high levels can lead to atherosclerosis.

HDL cholesterol protects against atherosclerosis through at least two mechanisms. First, HDL mediates the removal of excess cholesterol from peripheral tissues, such as blood vessels, and moves it back to the liver through a process known as reverse cholesterol transport. Once cholesterol is in the liver, it can be excreted from the body in bile. Therefore, higher levels of HDL allow for more excretion of excess cholesterol. Second, HDL impedes oxidation of LDL, which research suggests promotes atherosclerosis.

HDL levels are affected by androgens (testosterone) and in males are high before puberty. Athletes on anabolic steroids have HDL as low as 0.52 mmol/1. Peter's were 1.09–1.14 mmol/1 for many years (in spite of all the running which is supposed to elevate HDL). Now, since age 60, his value is 1.3 mmol/1, which he interprets as the effect of the decline in androgens. (There is a silver lining after all.)

The most dramatic effect of exercise on blood fats (lipids) is on triglycerides. This is an important effect because triglycerides are elevated in the metabolic abnormalities leading to insulin resistance and ultimately diabetes.

If your reading is over 200, you've got to make lifestyle changes to bring it down by limiting your intake of fat, particularly saturated animal fat, to no more than 30% of calories, a figure urged by the American Heart Association and other organisations.

A word for women: if you have high cholesterol and want to go on or stay on a birth-control pill, ask your doctor about formulations that can bring LDL down and raise HDL.

Have a blood pressure check. If it is high, you need to check it every year; if it's normal, every second year will be enough.

And, just in case, we recommend that you learn emergency procedures. Even better, have a table demonstrating emergency procedures handily placed – perhaps on the refrigerator. We hope you never have to use it, but knowledge of CPR and other crisis measures is part of the positive planning measures we advocate.

Reduce cancer risk

Cancer is the arch-enemy that most of us fear. Risk factors that are difficult to control are your genes and the environment in which you live, but your health habits play a role in determining whether you are a potential cancer victim.

If you are a smoker, make the next cigarette you stub out your last, because smoking is credited with being a leading cause of cancer, as well as heart disease. Stopping is an easy decision to make but surviving the withdrawal symptoms can be a tough hurdle for most of those who have pursued the cigarette habit heavily or for a long time. Fortunately, you and your willpower no longer need to be alone – your doctor can point you towards several nicotine-replacement therapies, such as nicotine gum, patches, nasal sprays and even an antidepressant, Zyban, which research suggests can minimise withdrawal symptoms, even if you are not depressed. Another reason for giving up is the effect of passive smoking on those around you. Peter lost his mother, Margaret Snell, who lived with a heavy smoker for 40 years, to lung cancer at age 90. It is likely that smoke inhalation from the environment around you will eventually cause problems.

Women over 18 years of age should have a regular check for cervical cancer, particularly if they are sexually active. The American Cancer Society advises that, between 20 and 40, women should have clinical breast examinations every three years; past 40, it should become a yearly event. Self-examination on a monthly basis should begin from the 20s, says Dr Susan Haas, chief of the Harvard Vanguard Division of Obstetrics and Gynecology at Brigham and Women's Hospital in Boston. 'Lumps that are especially worrisome feel like wood – not round, smooth and squishy like a grape,' she says.

If you're worried that you face the risk of breast cancer, you need to talk to your medical practitioner. He or she will know about

Tamoxifen, a drug which ongoing studies indicate may reduce that risk. But it could also introduce risks of its own because it has been linked to blood clotting in the lungs and veins and uterine cancer. At menopause, women at high risk of uterine cancer should have a sample of endometrial tissue examined for dysplasia (irregular cell growth that may be cancerous).

Beyond 50 years of age, both men and women should be checked every five years for colon and rectal cancer, and if small growths known as polyps are found, the physician will usually remove them and want to check more frequently. The American Cancer Society also recommends a flexible sigmoidoscopy every five years; or a colonoscopy or double-contrast barium enema every five to 10 years.

Once they reach 50, men should have a prostate-specific antigen (PSA) blood test and a digital rectal examination every year to screen for prostate cancer.

Cancer risk is higher when there is a family history. If you can, find out what those types of cancer were and tell your doctor. You could benefit from a more regular screening.

The work you do can pose threats to your health. Think about them and ask about them. Unsuspecting exposure to carcinogenic materials, such as asbestos, has shortened the lives of many people unnecessarily. Being unaware of the risk, they did nothing to protect themselves from insidious diseases, which sometimes do not materialise as illnesses until it is too late. The simple act of wearing a safety mask could have spared many workers.

Diabetes prevention

We have talked at length about diabetes. We reiterate that obesity is the greatest single cause of the type 2 diabetes, which makes it vital that you watch your weight constantly – it has the nasty habit of sneaking up on you – and your intake of sugary foods.

If you already have diabetes and are overweight, shedding only 5kg to 7kg can reduce symptoms and prevent some of the complications. Again, regular medical checks can give early warnings if you are at risk of diabetes. This could mean a fasting blood-glucose test at three-yearly intervals. If the figure is 3.27 mmol/1 or more, you are in the risk zone.

Have a simple blood test for glycosylated haemoglobin, which is used to measure blood-sugar control over an extended period. In normal individuals a small percentage of the haemoglobin (Hb) molecules in red blood cells becomes glycosylated (that is, chemically linked to glucose). The percentage of glycosylation is proportional to time and to concentration of glucose. In other words, older red blood cells will have a greater percentage of GHb and poorly controlled diabetics, with periods of time where they have high concentrations of blood glucose, will have a greater percentage of GHb.

Osteoporosis prevention

Osteoporosis, an increased risk for post-menopausal women, makes bones brittle and apt to break, but there may be ways of preventing it or at least staving it off. Bone mineral density tests can determine your risk factor. Hormone replacement therapy or a new designer oestrogen, raloxifene, are two possibilities but both could present other risk factors. Discuss this with your doctor.

Guard against skin cancer

The incidence of skin cancer is on the rise, yet it's one of the most preventable forms of cancer. People who spent their childhood summers bared to the sun without sunscreen protection cannot now escape the risk but everyone can minimise further damage. A sunscreen with a protection factor of at least 15 (preferably 30), applied on all exposed skin before you go outside, is advisable even if you plan to be out for only 10 minutes. Sun damage is cumulative.

Don't be fooled by those cloudy skies, either. The sun's rays still penetrate and harm the skin. Scotland is not noted for its excessive sunshine but was found some years ago to have one of the world's highest incidences of skin cancer.

The sun is a source of vitamin D – but you can get that from milk, which you can enjoy in the shade. Other excellent sources of vitamin D include fatty fish (salmon and herring), vitamin D-fortified milk, and egg yolks. However, the Cancer Council of Australia said in March

2005 that cancer specialists were rethinking the traditional advice to cover up in the sun because concern was growing that staying in the shade could be creating a vitamin D deficiency and increasing the risk of a range of diseases from rickets to osteoporosis.

Bruce Armstrong, professor of public health at Sydney University, said, 'It is a revolution. I have worked in public health and been preaching sun avoidance for 25 years. But what this statement says is that there are two sides to the story.'

The sun's action on the skin produces vitamin D, which can be stored by the body for up to 60 days. A shortage causes leg-deforming rickets in children and has also been linked to multiple sclerosis and diabetes. This is still a tenuous linkage and the real factor is that most people should limit sun exposure to avoid skin damage. If you think that the damage is insignificant, compare the skin on your forearms with the skin on your bum.

Peter has had multiple surgeries to remove skin cancers, which he attributes to his New Zealand heritage. Garth has had more than 40 surgical removals of various non-malignant but potentially dangerous skin lesions and many others burnt off.

Dermatologists are now arguing that the mantra that there is no such thing as a safe tan is wrong and the real problem is from sunburn, especially before the age of 20. Neil Walker, chairman of the UK Skin Cancer Prevention Working Party, has described warnings to avoid the sun entirely as draconian and unnecessary. He has the backing of Professor Brian Wharton, chairman of the British Nutrition Foundation, and Sara Hiom, head of health information at Cancer Research UK.

But, on the other side of this coin, the Auckland Cancer Society says 200 New Zealanders die every year from melanoma and people can get enough vitamin D simply by walking to the letterbox or the bus stop.

If the real enemy is sunburn, not simply exposure to the sun, then wide-brimmed hats, long pants and sleeves, as well as sunscreen, give the best protection. Not all fabrics have the same sun-screening properties and an ultraviolet protection factor scale for clothing has been published.

UPF ratings and protection categories

UPF rating	Protection category	% UVR blocked
15–24	Good	93.3–95.9
25–39	Very good	96.0–97.4
40 and over	Excellent	97.5 or more

The typical white cotton T-shirt so popular in summer is not your best bet. Its UPF rating is only seven, while dark–blue denim jeans are UPF 1000. Colour has an effect – for example, white polyester is 16 UPF, while black polyester is 34 UPF. We are in an age of apparent global warming and holes in the ozone layer, which are thought to intensify the sun's damaging habits. It's a pity but it's also a risk factor.

Sunglasses – and it has been found that the cheapest $12 darks are as good as the designer-labelled $200-plus ones – block 99 to 100% of both UVA and UVB light. Be careful that the glasses are effective in blocking UVA and UVB, otherwise dark glasses can actually cause the pupil to widen, thus permitting a larger amount of damaging UV rays to enter the eye. Prescription glasses should have the lenses covered with a clear coating that blocks UV.

Learn the facts about melanoma (cancerous skin tumours). Check your moles once-yearly in the mirror. Are they asymmetrical (one half of the mole doesn't match the other)? Are the borders notched, ragged, or blurred? Is the colour not uniform or intensely black? Is the diameter greater than six millimetres? If so, or if you notice something you think is questionable, see a dermatologist immediately. Catching cancer early could save your life.

Supercharge your diet

Your immunity to disease declines with age unless you take action, according to Jeffrey Blumberg, a professor of nutrition at Tufts University in Medford, Massachusetts.

To protect against high cholesterol, certain cancers and diabetes (among other serious health problems), get more fibre in your diet by eating plenty of whole grains, legumes, vegetables and fruit. Eat a varied diet to get all the vitamins and minerals you need.

Instead of fattier animal proteins (such as beef), eat more soy foods. Research suggests that tofu and other soy foods may reduce your risk of heart disease, certain cancers and osteoporosis, as well as reducing menopausal symptoms.

Men and women aged 19 to 50 are supposed to take 1000mg of calcium daily, 1200mg after age 50. But since most women don't get enough calcium from their diets, they should take a supplement, according to Dr Blumberg. Choose one that also contains vitamin D.

To protect against cancer, diabetes, heart disease and cataracts, take a multivitamin that contains 400µg of folic acid and a vitamin E supplement containing 100 to 400IU.

Don't overload on vitamins and minerals, though. Too much of some, such as vitamin B6 and vitamin A, can be dangerous.

Minimise stress

Stress is a term that is used to describe situations that cause certain emotional and physiological responses. Emotional stress occurs when you are worried about losing your job, or about having enough money to pay your bills, or about your mother if she needs an operation. In fact, to most of us, stress is synonymous with worry. If it is something that makes you worry, then it is stress.

As far as the body is concerned, the key condition is change. Anything that causes a change in your life causes stress. It doesn't matter if it is a 'good' change, or a 'bad' change, they are both stress. When you find your dream flat and get ready to move, that is stress. If you break your leg, that is stress. Good or bad, if it is a change in your life, it is stress as far as your body is concerned.

Chronic stress is unhealthy because it causes the release of hormones that constrict blood vessels and elevate blood pressure. As a positive influence, stress can help compel us to action; it can result in a new awareness and an exciting new perspective. As a negative influence, it can result in feelings of distrust, rejection, anger and depression, which in turn can lead to health problems such as headaches, upset stomach, rashes, insomnia, ulcers, high blood pressure, heart disease and stroke.

Classically, the primary physiological response to stress is 'fight or flight'. However, according to Shelley Taylor and her colleagues at UCLA, women's responses are more marked by a pattern of 'tend and befriend'. At the heart of this difference may be the hormone oxytocin, which is present in higher levels in women than men and released during stress. Oxytocin, when administered experimentally to animals, induces relaxation and reduces fearfulness and sympathetic activity. In women, oestrogen appears to enhance the effects whereas androgens inhibit oxytocin release.

An interesting connection with this hormone is its release during interaction of owners with their pets. This supports a study which found a better one-year survival after discharge from a coronary care unit in patients who had animal companions. Pets are more effective than spouses, possibly because they are generally more accepting of flaws in behaviour than spouses.

Here are some tips:

- Work to keep the friends you have, but make new ones, too. The more social connections you have, the better off your health may be.

- Be spiritual. Studies show that people involved in spiritual activities such as churchgoing tend to fare better healthwise, according to Dr Marty Sullivan, co-director of the Integrative Medicine Initiative at Duke University Medical Center in Durham, North Carolina. You can reap benefits by getting involved in something you care about deeply.

- Help others, but don't just donate money to charity. Studies show you'll derive health benefits only if you get personally involved.

- Don't skimp on sleep, or your ability to cope with stress will be impaired.

- Don't stay in a job you hate. Studies show that not liking your job can put you at risk for heart disease.

- Don't do too many things at once. Learn to prioritise your activities into an A (important), B (important but not critical) and C (not important) list. Do A things first, and reprioritise daily. Pace yourself. Your body and mind need time to rejuvenate.

Staying young

To maintain youthful stamina and energy, you *must* exercise. Without it, you'll lose 30 to 40% of your muscle mass between the ages of 30 and 70. Part of that exercise should be resistance-training because, as noted by Robert Butler, chief executive officer of the International Longevity Center at Mount Sinai Medical Center in New York City, aerobic exercise is not enough. Be sure to work all the major muscle groups in your arms, legs, and trunk.

Stretch *after* you exercise to prevent injury and stay flexible. Hold each stretch for 15 seconds without bouncing. If you intend to stretch before exercise, warm up first with light jogging or jogging on the spot — don't try to stretch cold muscles.

Expend at least 1000 calories a week exercising (the equivalent of walking briskly 5km a day, four times a week). Studies show, however, that even moderate physical activity increases longevity.

Studies of ageing cyclists (in their 60s and 70s) showed that, although reflexes do slow with age, they still had reaction times equivalent to inactive men in their 20s. One group of 70-year-olds, who had trained regularly from the age of 50, had a muscle cross-sectional area equivalent to a group of 28-year-old students. Without a regular exercise programme, a decrease in muscle mass from muscle fibre atrophy becomes particularly apparent at age 60 or thereabouts.

Aerobic capacity declines twice as fast in sedentary individuals and may even plateau with a regular training programme; the maximum heart rate does decline with age, and cardiac output falls. But a group of active 45-year-olds on a regular endurance exercise programme for 10 years was found to have maintained a stable blood pressure, body mass and VO_{2max} right through.

Cycling reasonable distances three or four times a week could mean you are 41% less likely to die from heart disease and 58% less likely to develop diabetes.

Caring for the brain

Where are my reading glasses? What have I come to buy from this shop? Who is that person? What's your name? Help, who am I? Perhaps it's not that serious yet, but fading or failing memory is a real problem of ageing and, again, it's something you can work to prevent.

It used to be thought that, each day, we lost thousands of the 100 billion neurons we had at birth. The good news is that we are not losing brain cells in significant numbers and that the older brain is capable of generating new cells.

The most reliably established effect of ageing is that older neurons process signals more slowly so that reaction time, the ability to retrieve information, perform complex tasks simultaneously or to learn new information are impaired. These changes may, in part, be genetic or result from the damaging effects of free radicals (unstable reactive molecules) which degrade the myelin sheath surrounding the long axons of nerve cells and slow signal transmission.

Risk factors for cognitive decline are:

- Atherosclerosis, which can decrease blood flow to the brain and cause 'mini strokes'.
- Alzheimer's disease – the apoE4 gene increases the risk.
- Exposure to neurotoxins, such as lead.
- Smoking, excess use of alcohol and mind–altering drugs.
- Lack of physical activity.
- Low level of mental activity.
- High stress levels.
- Depression.

Ten tips for a better brain:

1. Remain physically active – move it or lose it. Try activities that challenge the coordinating centres of the brain – for example, some of the balancing movements in t'ai chi.
2. Practise stress reduction by meditating, practising self-hypnotism or yoga.
3. Be socially active and have activities to look forward to.
4. Keep mentally active by working, doing puzzles, volunteering, taking on projects – use it or lose it again.
5. Use medication for damaging diseases such as hypertension, diabetes, depression, high cholesterol.
6. Use aids to assist impaired vision or hearing to help stay intellectually engaged. Many people with an increasing level of

deafness won't wear hearing aids. It's a matter of vanity, pride or a reluctance to accept a functional failure. So they move to the outside of social circles because they cannot adequately join in and, in time, become isolated.

7. Don't smoke.
8. Drink alcohol in moderation. Alcohol damages brain cells as well as livers.
9. Get adequate sleep.
10. Always have goals and think about them, plan them and revise them to keep your imagination alert. Think and ask yourself: what will you do when you have nothing left to do? Roll over and die? You should never run out of things you want to do; even if you never accomplish all of them, keeping them in mind and working towards them is a positive life-enhancing activity.

The conscious mind keeps one thought in the forefront and many others in the background with ready access. But if those thoughts are negative, they are constantly niggling away at the conscious edge. They are not beneficial thoughts. But, rather than trying to banish them, in line with a cognitive therapy approach, try reformulating them.

For example, rather than thinking 'I always get things wrong', which, invariably, is definitely not the case, it is better to think 'sometimes I get things wrong, but often I get it right'.

One man's stress is another man's challenge. Obstacles are what you see when you take your eye off the goal. This is fairly straightforward positive thinking – the 'glass is half-full' approach instead of the 'glass is half-empty'.

Worrying about things we cannot control is one of the great stress factors. Worry will not cure anything. But, except perhaps for raging optimists, it's a difficult frame of mind to overcome.

However, the very process of training yourself to give up worrying about matters beyond your control may, in itself, be a valuable mental exercise.

Mental health

Widen your range of activities; this will improve the connection between nerve cells that relay messages in the brain. It is that loss of connection that leaves you wondering what you're supposed to be doing or unable to recall what you set out to do a few minutes ago. For example, if you work with figures, you might spend some of your spare time doing ceramics, writing or painting to protect against mental decline.

When you need to do some mathematical task, such as balancing your cheque book or adding up a list of shopping prices, don't grab the calculator – we are assuming that you can remember where you left it – but do it in your head. It may take a little longer but it will also help you to keep your collection of memory marbles intact a little longer.

Foods that are high in the antioxidant vitamins, such as C, E (found in nuts) and beta-carotene (found in red, yellow and orange fruit and vegetables) are thought to protect cells in the brain responsible for memory by blocking the attack of free radicals on the cell's DNA. So eat plenty. They cannot do you any harm and they could be doing you a power of good.

Physical exercise protects your brain as it ages

Physical exercise has a protective effect on the brain and its mental processes, and may even help prevent Alzheimer's disease. Exercise and health data from a study of nearly 5000 men and women over 65 years of age found that those who exercised were less likely to lose their mental abilities or develop dementia, including Alzheimer's.

Furthermore, the five-year study, at the Laval University in Sainte-Foy, Quebec, suggests that the more you exercise the greater the protective benefits for the brain, particularly if you are a woman.

Inactive individuals were twice as likely to develop Alzheimer's, compared with those with the highest levels of activity (vigorous exercise at least three times a week). But even light or moderate exercisers cut their risk significantly for Alzheimer's and mental decline, according to a report in the *Archives of Neurology* in March 2001.

So how does physical exercise help the brain to stay young? Quite simply, exercise improves cardiovascular health, which increases the flow of oxygen-rich blood to the brain. Over a lifetime, this makes a big difference to brain function. In fact, cardiovascular health appears to be the primary biological reason why elderly women tend to have better cognitive function than men.

When Dutch researchers tested 600 people aged 85 and over, they found that the odds of having a better memory were 80% higher in women, even after considering factors such as formal education and depression. 'Good cognitive speed was found in 33% of the women and 28% of the men,' they reported.

Women at age 85 are known to be relatively free from cardiovascular disease, compared to men, and this relative absence of atherosclerosis is a likely biological explanation for better brain function.

What's heart smart is brain gain

Psychologist James Blumenthal underlines the long-term importance of exercise for brain function: 'We know that, in general, exercise improves the heart's ability to pump blood more effectively, as well as increasing the blood's oxygen-carrying capacity. It is thought that one of the reasons why the elderly – especially those with coronary artery disease or hypertension – tend to suffer some degree of cognitive decline is in part due to a reduction in blood flow to the brain.'

Blumenthal and a team of researchers at Duke University Medical Center found that an aerobic exercise programme decreased depression and improved the cognitive abilities of middle-aged and elderly men and women.

They followed 156 patients, between the ages of 50 and 77, who had been diagnosed with major depressive disorder. They were randomly assigned to one of three groups: exercise, medication, or a combination of medication and exercise. The exercise group spent 30 minutes either riding a stationary bicycle or walking or jogging three times a week.

The researchers were surprised to find that, after 16 weeks, all three groups showed statistically significant and identical improvements in standard measurements of depression, implying that exercise was just as effective as medication in treating major depression.

Before enrolling in the trial, and four months later, the cognitive abilities of the participants were tested in four areas: memory, executive functioning, attention/concentration, and psychomotor speed.

Compared to the medication group, the exercisers showed significant improvements in the higher mental processes of memory and in 'executive functions' that involve planning, organisation and the ability to mentally juggle different intellectual tasks at the same time.

'What we found so fascinating was that exercise had its beneficial effect in specific areas of cognitive function that are rooted in the frontal and prefrontal regions of the brain,' says Blumenthal. 'The implications are that exercise might be able to offset some of the mental declines that we often associate with the ageing process.'

Blood sugar and exercise

Diabetes is a serious threat to the brain, so long-term blood sugar control is important to mental function. An analysis of more than a dozen studies comparing the effects of exercise versus no exercise showed that regular exercise significantly lowered the blood glucose levels in 528 adults with type 2 diabetes. They trained aerobically or with weights and may or may not have lost weight according to the American Diabetes Association annual meeting in June 2001.

Ongoing animal studies at the Salk Institute show that running can boost brain cell survival in mice that have a neurodegenerative disease with properties similar to Alzheimer's.

When these mice were sedentary, it appeared that most newly born brain cells died. The researchers did not understand that fully, but it probably had something to do with an inability to cope with oxidative stress. Running appeared to rescue many of these cells that would otherwise die.

Significantly, the miles logged correlated directly with the numbers of increased cells, almost as if the mice were wearing pedometers. Those that ran more grew more cells.

Running's brain-boosting effects were in the hippocampus, a region of the brain linked to learning and memory and known to be affected by Alzheimer's disease, which suggested that exercise might delay the onset and progression of some neurodegenerative diseases.

This study built on earlier work showing that running also leads to increased brain cell numbers in normal adult mice, elderly 'senior citizen' mice, and a genetically 'slow-learning' strain of mice. The studies have shown that new cell growth occurs in human brains, too. Therefore, this suggests that the boosting effects of running occurs in people as well.

Animal studies show that intellectual enrichment can even compensate for some forms of physical brain damage. For example, a mentally stimulating environment helped protect rats from the potentially damaging effects of lead poisoning.

Neuroscientists at Jefferson Medical College compared groups of rats given lead-laced water for several weeks in two different environments. Rats living in a stimulating environment showed a better ability to learn compared to the animals that were isolated. Behaviourally, living in an enriched environment seemed to help protect their brains. The magnitude of the protective effect was surprising and could lead to an early educational intervention for at-risk populations to diminish the damage that lead does to children by manipulating their socio-behavioural environment.

From an evolutionary point of view, it seems that the brain's ability to rewire its circuitry and repair itself after injury became the same mechanism it used to construct memories. Since both memory and repair depend on stimulation, this makes mental challenge an obvious and vital component of maintaining memory throughout life.

A matter of mood swings

Research into the interaction between ageing and exercise has thrown up some interesting and sometimes controversial theories. But all investigations seem to suggest that exercise as you grow older can only be good for you.

One study, focusing on the effect of exercise on mood in an elderly population of men and women, determined that, while exercise improved mood, it had no long-lasting effects if it was stopped. To reap the beneficial effects of exercise, exercise had to continue. The study confirmed earlier research but it showed that people who had exercised in the 1980s and stopped in the following decade lost the mood-enhancing benefits of exercise.

The study involved 944 residents of the northern San Diego County community of Rancho Bernardo during two time periods, 1984–87 and 1992–95. In the 1980s the residents – all physically able men and women aged between 50 and 89 – exercised at least three times a week. Their mood, measured by the Beck Depression Inventory (BDI), indicated that they generally had a healthy mood with no evidence of depression.

The same individuals were followed in the 1990s. Those still exercising continued to have low BDI scores, indicating a more positive mood and general well-being. But the BDI scores of those no longer exercising had risen to levels similar to residents who had never exercised during the two-decade study. The study determined that the increased age of the individuals was not a factor.

The study also found that a group of elderly residents who had not exercised in the 1980s, but began exercise in the 1990s had a less depressed mood and scores similar to those who were exercising through both study periods.

The study results were considered somewhat unexpected because it had been thought there could be a chance that people who exercised in the past would retain a level of enhanced mood, or lower depression, even though they no longer exercised.

A look on the downside

With all these fantastic benefits associated with regular exercise, perhaps we should also consider whether there are any negatives to regular exercise.

For example, many individuals say they exercise to a 'look and feel good' concept. But it seems that exercise, with all its many benefits, can also increase the formation of the dangerous free radicals associated with many disease-related health conditions. An acute bout of strenuous physical exercise may pose an oxidant insult to the heart. However, despite some discrepancies in the literature, there is a general trend showing that chronic regular physical exercise may beneficially influence cardiac antioxidant defences and promote overall cardiac function.

Free radicals are highly reactive and unstable molecules that can cause cellular damage. They are constantly formed in the human body by normal metabolism and are also created from other sources such as radiation, cigarette smoke and air pollution as listed below:

- tobacco smoke
- air pollution
- rancid dietary fats
- radiation (all forms)
- herbicides, pesticides, insecticides
- poor nutrition
- inflammatory diseases
- increased intake of polyunsaturated fats, which become unstable when heated
- alcohol and caffeine

Free radicals are known to damage cell membranes, proteins and DNA. Under normal conditions, the body has an efficient system to keep these free radicals in check. The body uses antioxidants to attack these free radicals and render them harmless before they can wreak havoc, but exercise is not what we would call normal conditions.

As you exercise, the body's demand for energy increases, which increases the body's use of oxygen, glucose and fats. According to Lester Packer, renowned expert on antioxidants, 'there is a delicate balance between oxidants (free radicals) and antioxidants, yet exercise, like disease, can tip the balance toward excessive free radical production'.

The solution is to tip the balance back the other way by increasing your consumption of antioxidants. This is not as challenging as it may sound because antioxidants are easily obtained. Food sources include red-, yellow-, green- or orange-coloured fruit and vegetables, and unrefined oils, brewer's yeast and whole grains. In essence, if you concentrate on an adequate and regular supply of the right foods, you will achieve an excellent supply of antioxidants. If you cannot follow that regimen every day, supplements may be the answer.

Antioxidants come in many forms, including vitamins, minerals and herbs. Some of the more important antioxidants include vitamin E (natural vitamin E is five times more effective than synthetic vitamin E), vitamin C, beta-carotene and selenium.

There is also exciting new research on co-enzyme Q10 and alpha-lipoic acid. CoQ10 plays a vital role in energy production and works with vitamin E as a primary fat-soluble antioxidant. Alpha-lipoic acid is called the 'universal antioxidant' because it is both fat- and water-soluble, meaning it can fight free radicals both inside and outside the cell. It also has the ability to reactivate both vitamins E and C once they have been used to fight free radicals.

Each antioxidant counteracts specific types of free radicals, which makes it important to provide your body with a variety. Most multivitamin and mineral formulas contain the major antioxidants. With the new research surrounding antioxidants, it is easy to find quality antioxidant formulas that provide a full spectrum of valuable antioxidant protection.

A pain in the back

A regular exercise programme has recognised benefits even for people who may be deterred by such conditions as joint pain, back pain, arthritis or osteoporosis, or who are recovering from an injury or surgery such as joint replacement or arthroscopy. Exercise has also been shown to benefit, at any age, by helping to lower blood pressure, reduce the risks of falls and serious injuries (such as hip or wrist fractures) and slow the body's loss of muscle and bone mass. Here are some of those ways in which exercise helps:

- Increases flexibility.
- Tones muscles.
- Builds stronger bones.
- Improves mobility and balance.
- Boosts self-image.
- Relieves insomnia.
- Relieves tension and stress.
- Maintains a healthy weight.

- Enhances cardiovascular fitness.
- Controls appetite.
- Increases HDL cholesterol levels.
- Reduces the risk of disease (e.g., diabetes).
- Provides fun and enjoyment.
- Provides for a longer, healthier life.
- Reduces joint and muscle pain.

With today's medical technology and scientific advances, the average life expectancy for men and women is increasing. It was revealed in 2005 that New Zealand men and women have recorded the largest improvement in life expectancy in the developed world during the past decade.

New Zealand men who reach the age of 60 can expect to live to 80 and women at 60 can expect to reach 84, according to a report on 22 member countries in the Organisation for Economic Cooperation and Development (OECD). This finding moved New Zealand from 20th ranking to 13th.

People are also looking for a higher quality of life – with greater importance placed on independent, healthy living. Exercise is a great way to keep older people active, but should be approached with caution. Exercise doesn't have to be vigorous to be beneficial.

As many gerontologists and researchers have found, exercise is the closest thing to an anti-ageing pill that exists. People who are physically fit, eat a healthy, balanced diet and take nutritional supplements can measure out to be 10 to 20 years younger biologically than their chronological age. This is what makes an immortal. An immortal doesn't necessarily live for ever but can be free from mental and physical disease and degeneration for years longer than an unhealthy individual. Exercise is an extremely important part of achieving this 'immortality'.

It doesn't matter if you were once physically active in your younger years. If you're not currently engaged in a physical activity programme on a regular basis, your body is not receiving the innumerable health-related benefits of exercise:

- Improves immune system functioning.

- Helps you lose weight – especially fat.
- Improves survival rate from heart attack.
- Improves body posture.
- Reduces risk of heart disease.
- Improves the body's ability to use fat for energy during physical activity.
- Helps the body resist upper respiratory tract infections.
- Helps relieve the pain of tension headaches.
- Increases maximal oxygen uptake.
- Increases muscle strength.
- Helps preserve lean body tissue.
- Reduces risk of developing high blood pressure.
- Increases density and breaking strength of ligaments and tendons.
- Improves coronary artery circulation.
- Increases levels of HDL cholesterol and reduces LDL cholesterol.
- Helps improve short-term memory.
- Sharpens dynamic vision and controls glaucoma.
- Reduces risk of developing type 2 diabetes.
- Reduces anxiety.
- Assists in quitting smoking.
- Slows the rate of joint degeneration (osteoarthritis).
- Enhances sexual desire, performance and satisfaction.
- Helps in the management of stress.
- Improves quality of sleep.
- Reduces risk of developing colon cancer.
- Reduces risk of developing prostate cancer.
- Reduces risk of developing breast cancer.
- Reduces risk of developing stroke.
- Reduces susceptibility to coronary thrombosis (a clot in the artery that supplies the heart with blood).
- Helps alleviate depression.
- Helps alleviate lower-back pain.
- Improves mental alertness and reaction time.
- Improves physical appearance.
- Improves self-esteem.

- Decreases resting heart rate.
- Helps in relaxation.
- Helps prevent and relieve the stresses that cause carpal tunnel syndrome.
- Helps relieve constipation.
- Protects against 'creeping obesity' – slow weight gain that occurs with age.
- Improves blood circulation, resulting in better-functioning organs, including the brain.
- Increases productivity at work.
- Improves balance and coordination.
- Helps to retard bone loss, thereby reducing your risk of developing osteoporosis.
- Improves general mood.
- Helps in maintaining an independent lifestyle.
- Increases overall health awareness.
- Improves overall quality of life.

If you are not convinced by these benefits, read the list again but substitute the positive verbs such as 'helps', 'reduces' and 'improves' with the negatives 'hinders', 'increases' and 'lessens'. Then you have to be convinced.

Mental gymnastics

That's rather a broad-brush reaction to a study led by an exercise physiologist at the Cleveland Clinic Foundation in Ohio, Dr Guang Yue. It's a long way from sprawling on the couch in front of the TV and thinking you should be taking some exercise.

The muscle Dr Yue and his colleagues began working on was the one that moves the little finger sideways. Subjects who visualised exercising that finger increased the strength of that specific muscle. So he set 10 volunteers, aged 20 to 35, to imagine flexing one of their biceps as hard as possible in training sessions five times a week. No cheating was allowed – the researchers recorded electrical brain activity during the sessions but also monitored the electrical impulses at the motor neurons, or nerve cells, of their arm muscles to make sure they were not, intentionally or unintentionally, tensing.

After a few weeks biceps strength was up 13.5% and the gain was maintained for three months after the training stopped.

If the technique works in older people, they might be able to use it to maintain strength and it could help patients too weak for exercise to begin recuperating from strokes or other injuries. So Dr Yue and his team have turned their attention to a group aged 65 to 80 to see if mental gymnastics also works for them.

There is some precedent for this remarkable discovery. Hull University sports psychologist Dr Peter Clough says it is well known that merely visualising playing a sport can often be a more effective way of getting better at it than actually practising. This may be a small ray of hope for the golf hacker – think hard enough about playing a round in two over par and maybe it will happen.

However, Dr Clough warns that muscle strength is just one aspect of taking exercise. Flexibility and aerobic quality are important and cannot be achieved by concentrated thought.

He doesn't think sitting on a sofa thinking about exercising a specific muscle group is really a good idea – and neither do we. Simply building muscle mass might make you look good but that is not what exercise is all about. To be effective, exercise has to raise the heart rate to 70% of its maximum for 20 minutes three times a week – that is what will help you to live longer better. There is no evidence that you can 'think' your heart rate to do that.

It is clear that there are individual differences in responsiveness to training. Not all athletes doing the same training under the same coach will make the Olympics. One genetic difference is muscle fibre type. If you have a preponderance of fast-twitch fibres, you will make a better sprinter than the person dominated by slow-twitch fibres. That person, again depending on the balance, may make a great marathon runner or middle-distance runner. However, there will be an improvement in fitness among sedentary people provided the training stimulus reaches a moderate intensity threshold.

We make this observation following an ABC News story, which suggested that some people will not respond to the stimulus of exercise at all. Unfortunately, the story discussed flawed research published in the *Journal of Applied Physiology* in 1999 under the title 'Familial aggregation of VO_{2max} response to exercise training: results from the HERITAGE family study'. Claude Bouchard was the lead author of this study in which heart rate-controlled cycle ergometers were used. The problem was that in older subjects the heart rate is not as responsive as in younger subjects and a brief amount of heavy work was required to get the heart rate into the 'training zone'. Thereafter the power output declined markedly even though the heart rate remained on target. Thus it was likely that this reduction in exercise dose was the cause of approximately 85 of their 481 subjects achieving a minimal training effect.

Many of Peter's colleagues have also criticised this study. His guess is that the reviewers may have spotted the problem with the heart rate criterion but didn't want to reject the paper because of the interesting genetic analysis. The story suggested that people's genes may determine their benefit from exercise, but to suggest that some don't respond at all to training is highly unlikely. There is no doubt that the degree of response to training is widely varied – a perfect example of this is all the Lydiard runners of Peter's era who worked as hard as Murray Halberg, Barry Magee and Peter did but didn't make it to the Olympics. Though several of them were among Lydiard athletes who for years divided up all the New Zealand national distance-running titles between them to the exclusion of their rivals who didn't put in the same effort.

Another aspect to this particular example is that, until Peter and the others training with Lydiard came under the Lydiard influence, none would have been regarded as prospective Olympians. However, it was assumed that they all had some kind of 'special talent' that Lydiard had been lucky enough to exploit. This, of course, was also pretty stupid. Physically, they were an odd assortment with no readily identifiable similarities that might have led to the special talent label. It was they who were lucky to come under the influence of Lydiard and, in the process of becoming a highly successful team of runners, they underscored the theory we now expound: that anyone, given the right encouragement and exercise, can improve beyond all expectations.

How can a person be motivated to exercise?

Fewer than 10% of adults exercise at least four times a week and more than half quit within six months of starting an exercise programme. The same problems hold true for children. Experts state that children should be physically active for at least 60 minutes per day or longer, if possible. Children are born motivated for physical action.

Why, then, have people stopped moving? With so many high-tech computer and video games to distract them, children seem averse to old-fashioned exercises like running around on the playground or clambering up a jungle gym. Parents and guardians may also find it hard to make time for an evening jog or a game of catch with the kids when interesting programmes are on television or a good movie is playing just around the corner. If both parents are working, the problem seems to be compounded.

Adults must make conscious efforts to oppose these cultural pressures, not only for themselves, but for their children. Even children who aren't interested in joining a sports team may enjoy a round of catch with their parents, walking in the park, or swimming.

Early school physical education programmes can make a significant difference and the earlier these routines are learned, the more likely they will be carried forward into a healthy adulthood. Unfortunately, many schools equate physical health only with athletic success, discouraging participation in athletic activities by everyone except a few talented individuals.

And, after graduation, athletically gifted youngsters often fail to continue training once they lose the encouragement of coaches and fans, their only gauge of self-worth. Studies have shown that people tend to give up more quickly and feel less competent if their perceptions of success are based on comparison to their peers rather than team cooperation or individual improvement and self-mastery.

Success in competition is often not within a person's control. People mature at different rates, and there seems to be a genetic component to coordination, strength, speed and one's response to resistance exercise. Nonetheless, everyone should strive to be as fit as they possibly can within the limitations of their strengths.

Unfortunately, weight loss is the greatest motivator to exercise for women and muscle tone is the primary motivator for men. Such cosmetic effects may take a long time to become apparent, discouraging people from continuing even though their health is improving. Much more important should be the health benefits exercise has for everyone. How you look is not as important as how you feel.

Another deterrent to exercise is the perception of an unending sameness. Jog, jog, jog, or lift, lift, lift. It has been suggested that, instead of thinking of exercise as a 'diet', one should think of it as a 'menu', with many exciting and pleasurable offerings.

New studies show that cross-training, regularly switching from one type of exercise to another, is more beneficial than focusing only on one form of exercise. You don't need to endure long, dreary workouts, because it is possible to choose physical activities that are enjoyable, such as sports, dancing or biking. Exercising with other people or developing an interest or hobby that requires physical activity is likely to make an otherwise arduous routine much more pleasant.

Sticking to a prepared schedule and recording one's progress can be strong motivators. Research shows that older adults adhere very well to a home-based exercise programme that includes videotapes and motivational support from health professionals. Experts assert that even a little bit of advice and discussion with a family doctor can help spur on sedentary patients.

And everyone can adopt simple changes in daily routine, like climbing the stairs instead of taking the elevator, walking instead of driving to the local dairy, or canoeing instead of zooming along in a powerboat. Even small efforts can boost fitness levels and lay the groundwork for a healthy lifestyle.

Final reminders on how to use it and not lose it

These activities are especially beneficial when performed regularly, according to your age and fitness level:

- Brisk walking, hiking, stair-climbing, any aerobic exercise.

- Jogging, running, skating, cycling, rowing and swimming.
- Activities such as soccer and basketball that include continuous movement.

The training effects of such activities are most apparent at exercise intensities that exceed 5% of a person's exercise capacity (maximum heart rate). If you're physically active regularly for longer periods or at greater intensity, you're likely to benefit more. But don't overdo it.

For people who can't exercise vigorously or who are sedentary, even moderate-intensity activities, when performed daily, can have some long-term health benefits. They help lower the risk of cardio-vascular diseases. Here are some examples:

- Walking for pleasure, gardening and yard work.
- Housework, dancing and prescribed home exercise.
- Recreational activities such as tennis, soccer, basketball and touch football.

These need not be high-intensity activities if you indulge in them with peer groups with similar levels of fitness.

When should I consult my doctor?

If any or all of these benefits inspire you, look before you leap (or lurch) out of your chair and go to find some gear to exercise in. You should always consult your doctor before you start a vigorous exercise programme. Explain what you want to do and get him or her to check you over to see if any of these apply to you:

- During or right after you exercise, you often have pains or pressure in the left or mid-chest area, left neck, shoulder or arm.
- You have a heart condition or you've had a stroke, and your doctor recommended only medically supervised physical activity.
- You've developed chest pain or discomfort within the last month.
- You tend to lose consciousness or fall due to dizziness.
- You feel extremely breathless after mild exertion.
- Your doctor recommended you take medicine for your blood

pressure, a heart condition or a stroke.

- Your doctor said you have bone, joint or muscle problems that could be made worse by some forms of physical activity.
- You have a medical condition or other physical reason not mentioned here that may need special attention in an exercise programme (for example, insulin-dependent diabetes).
- You're middle-aged or older, haven't been physically active, and plan a relatively vigorous exercise programme.

If none of these apply to you, or your medical professional gives you the green light, you can start on a gradual, sensible programme of increased activity tailored to your needs. If you feel any of the physical symptoms listed above when you start your exercise programme, contact your doctor right away. If one or more of the above is true for you, an exercise-stress test may be used to help plan a safe and beneficial exercise programme.

So, do we as ageing authors do, practise what we preach. We'll let you be the judges.

Peter Snell closes in on three score and ten

As I look back over my life, various milestones can be neatly packaged into decades. The first two representing the First Age of dependence, the second to fifth decades, being the Second Age of the career builder and provider, to finally beyond 50 years, the Third Age, which is the subject of this book. For me the first decade involved the innocence of growing up in the seaside town of Opunake. There was a lot of clambering around the cliffs, frolicking in the heavy surf and in general laying the foundation for a physically active life.

The second decade saw the family move to the bigger, but still small, town of Te Aroha which was nestled at the foot of a 952m mountain that provided ample opportunity for teenage adventure. These were the years when the foundation of sporting skills was laid, including rugby, tennis, badminton, golf, cricket, hockey, gymnastics and even running. The decade was not one of academic achievement and at the age of 19 I was faced with selecting a career path that did not require university education. It was at this time that a major life-changing decision was made to abandon ball games and explore my abilities as a runner.

The decision paid off and the third decade was dominated by athletic achievement. New Zealand championships at the mile and 880 yards at 20 and an Olympic gold medal at 21 were followed by world records, British Commonwealth gold and more Olympic gold at Tokyo. This decade was also most notable for family – my marriage to first wife Sally and the birth of two daughters, Amanda and Jacqueline.

I like to see the fourth decade as one of maturity and reaching a critical decision point in my life – accept my safe, comfortable but somewhat unsatisfying existence or risk it all and boldly strike out in a new direction. The 'mid-life crisis' came at the age of 34 when I decided that the only way to lift myself into a satisfying career was to acquire academic qualifications. With Sally's agreement our house in Auckland was sold and we moved to Davis, California, where I enrolled at the University of California, to major in human performance. The decade concluded within a year of completing my PhD at the Department of Physical Education at Washington State University.

In the fifth decade the challenge was to translate seven years of formal education into a satisfying career and this was accomplished via a post-doctoral fellowship and later faculty position at the University of Texas Southwestern Medical Center, where I engaged in exercise-related research and had responsibility for a faculty/staff wellness programme. My marriage to Sally ended when I left California for Washington State, and in Texas I met my second wife, Miki, a talented runner in her own right.

During the sixth decade health and fitness issues were important. Miki and I embraced the sport of orienteering which provided us with competitive opportunities as runners but with the interesting twist of map-reading and navigation. We both became aware of declining fitness combined with the need for magnifying glasses to read and the development of arthritic pain in various parts of the body, the knees, and in my case, a stiff shoulder arising from multiple sports injuries.

Today as I approach the end of the seventh decade, I am following the advice given in this book by keeping busy at work but not so busy that I do not have time to spend with Miki travelling, cycling and working out together. Miki does Curves three times per week and often accompanies me part of the way on my 13km bike ride to work. Our running has given way to a combination of walking and jogging for 3km to 5km. Activities that might once have been considered chores such as mowing lawns and garden maintenance are now seen as 'exercise opportunities'. Miki keeps busy with a variety of artistic endeavours. We both spend time on our computers managing finances and paying bills online; Miki also writes a monthly orienteering newsletter. To keep the mind active we do crosswords and I am not beyond playing video games that demand thinking ahead or sharp hand-eye coordination. I try to do something every day that challenges the cardiovascular system and muscles, as well as stretching to maintain a good range of motion. Push-ups, leg-lifts and sit-ups are among the easiest floor exercises and have great benefits. I see a dentist every three to six months, to maintain the health of my teeth and gums, and visit a doctor every other year. My total cholesterol is low at 8mmol/1, triglycerides at 38mmol/1 and HDL cholesterol at 2.7mmol/1. My blood pressure is 125/75 but rises with stress, which I try to control. My preventive approach to cancer is a six-monthly visit to the dermatologist, a colonoscopy every five years and a bi-yearly test for prostate-specific antigen (PSA). My diet is fairly normal other than trying to limit high-glycaemic carbohydrates and using artifical sweetener in my tea (I have never enjoyed the taste of coffee). Occasionally I will have a glass of Marlborough wine, a beer on hot weekends, and once a week a frozen Margarita, invented here in Dallas. I take an antioxidant containing 500mg of vitamin C, 400mg of vitamin E, 25,000 IU beta-carotene and 50mcg of selenium (immune function support). This year I passed on having a flu shot.

It is my objective to do research at UT Southwestern until I am at least 70 and stay as mentally active as possible in retirement. Golf, cycling (mountain bikes), orienteering and one game of racquetball a week fulfil my dose of healthy exercise.

Peter Snell
Dallas, Texas
December 2005

Garth Gilmour faces the eighth decade

The approach of 80 years of age opens new doors in the mind to release intriguing, fresh scenarios. It's a balancing process between the realisation that, this far past the traditional three score and ten, I could drop dead at any minute without warning – I knew people who have done that – or I could fall victim to some ailment that takes an interminable time to kill me. I could go on for another 10 years. Or 20. Even, as my doctor once said in a burst of enthusiasm, another 40.

I am the same age as the Queen, who seems fairly indestructible. If I make 100, will she still be around to send me a congratulatory message? I would enjoy sending one back.

Life is finite, with widely variable conditions attached that determine the point at which the finite point is established. So there is no sense in worrying about it.

All that aside, what shape am I in at 80?

Well, I am aware – at times sharply reminded – of aches, pains and twinges that have recently introduced themselves, unasked, into my daily life. I have, fortunately, a high pain tolerance honed on an excruciating spinal episode in the early 1970s following years of intermittent agonies in my lower back, so I can handle this nagging motley of lesser discomforts. I also have a relaxed philosophical approach to life, developed in the 20 years since bowel cancer was discovered and excised, leaving behind only the occasional thought that it might, one day, return. No good can come of worrying about that either.

My knees are my worst problem. They are one legacy of a late burst of long-distance running from the age of 35 into my late 50s but they actually act for me as a reminder that if I hadn't become a runner I would probably have been dead long ago. I have often said that I owe my longevity to joining forces with the wonderful Arthur Lydiard, who turned me almost overnight, at our first meeting, from a smoking, drinking, unfit journalist into a jogger and then a marathon runner. He led me – or shamed me – to an existence that proved to be pure joy after the hungover, coughing, head-sore and limiting life I was leading.

Everyone should have an Arthur Lydiard in their lives. I have been doubly fortunate; I am also in a happy, contented marriage with a fitness-aware woman who can walk the legs off me.

I solved the knee problem easily enough by going back to the bicycle as a way of keeping physically and mentally fit. I had ridden track in Wanganui in my early 20s, and once you have ridden a bike you never forget how not to fall off. Being knocked off is another matter but I have survived those episodes with no more than blood loss, bruises and some stitches.

I have been a casual cycle trainer, as I was for most of my running years, but I maintained a fitness sufficient to get me round the worst 100km of a 160km ride round Lake Taupo in the central North Island of New Zealand in 2003. I cover a lot of miles on a racer on rollers indoors because it saves me time. And skin and blood.

Most summers I have swum fairly regularly and made it a goal to cover the length of my local beach (about 1km) before the season ends. My wife Kay, a diligent walker at 75, swims even more regularly and a year or two back was in the sea every day of the calendar year (no wetsuit but the enticement of a monetary reward if she succeeded).

When I'm not in front of my computer, which is where I am seven days a week but at times that suit me, I work outside, which can involve mowing a large expanse of lawn, digging and tending several patches of garden and, when the opportunity arises and my wife encourages me, clearing out some of the trees that have grown too large for the place in the past three decades. I am very happy high up in a tree with my chainsaw.

I am equally happy with crossword puzzles, both standard and cryptic, as a mental activity and read as much as I can when I can. I tend to devour the daily newspaper from front to back. I am also secretary-treasurer of an association of 32 community boards scattered across the upper North Island.

My concession to the physical degradation of 80 years has been to keep doing everything I always did but at a slower pace and in shorter bursts.

I do 150-plus crunches and 35-plus push-ups four to six times a week and employ some of the simple isometric exercises contained in this book. There are times when I miss a few days but my conscience always stabs me back to a semblance of commitment and regularity.

I visit a chiropractor once a month and she relieves my tight shoulders and sore neck and sends me off feeling about 60.

My resting heart rate is 58, my blood pressure is that of a 25-year-old and my weight, at just over 68kg, is much the same as it was when I was 20, 30, 40, 50, 60 and 70, notwithstanding the variable lifestyle I have pursued during those decades. My golf, which, like everything else, tends to be spasmodic, is not greatly worse than it was when I played fairly regularly some 40 to 50 years ago.

I hope that if I reach 100 I will be able to break 100 on a golf course. It would be nice to play to my age and, of course, the odds improve in my favour with every year that passes. When I was 30, I was about 50 shots away from that target; now I am only about 10 away.

Maybe that marks what may well be my greatest asset – optimism, coupled with the fact that I never worry about anything, least of all what my future has in store for me. I am too busy enjoying today to be concerned about tomorrow.

I never feel that I am now 80. I don't feel particularly old and, from my perspective, Peter Snell and Kay are still youngsters.

What I enjoy least in life is watching my peers letting themselves go. I am aware of what they are doing: surrendering to their advancing years without a fight.

Garth Gilmour
Milford, Auckland
December 2005

And a final thought

We began this book with Shakespeare's famous 'seven ages' poem, an elegant exercise in witty but thought-provoking observation. We close it with a modern poem with equal wit and insight:

The ages of success

At age 4, success is . . . not peeing your pants

At age 12, success is . . . having friends

At age 16, success is . . . having a driver's licence

At age 20, success is . . . having sex

At age 35, success is . . . having money

At age 50, success is . . . having money

At age 60, success is . . . having sex

At age 70, success is . . . having a driver's licence

At age 75, success is . . . having friends

At age 80, success is . . . not peeing your pants

Acknowledgements

When writing this book we consulted the work of the following people involved in the research of ageing and physical health: William Aronson, Jonsson Cancer Center and UCLA Department of Physiological Science, California; Carrolee Barlow, The Salk Institute for Biological Studies, California; Michael Blumenthal, Duke University, North Carolina; Dr Robert Butler, International Longevity Center at Mt Sinai Medical Center, New York; Richard Restak, Laval University, Quebec; Jay Schneider, Jefferson Medical College, Philadelphia; Dr Nicola Scopinaro, University of Genoa, Genoa; Dr George Vaillant, Harvard Medical School, Massachusetts; Molly Wagster, National Institute of Aging, Maryland; Dr West, Men's Health Information and Resource Centre, University of Western Sydney, New South Wales.

References

Allen K, Blascovich J, Mendes WB. 'Cardiovascular reactivity and the presence of pets, friends and spouses: the truth about cats and dogs'. *Psychosomatic Medicine*. 2002; 64(5): 727–39.

Centers for Disease Control and Prevention and American College of Sports Medicine Physical Activity and Public Health. 'A recommendation from the Centers for Disease Control and Prevention and the American College of Sports Medicine'. *Journal of the American Medical Association*. 1995; 273: 402–7.

Child JS, Barnard RJ, Taw TL. 'Cardiac hypertrophy and function in Master endurance runners and sprinters'. *Journal of Applied Physiology: Respiratory, Environmental & Exercise Physiology*. 1984; 57: 176–81.

Committee on Exercise, Rehabilitation, and Prevention, Council on Clinical Cardiology, American Heart Association. 'Resistance exercise in individuals with and without cardiovascular disease. Benefits, rationale, safety, and prescription'. *Circulation*. 2000; 101: 828–33.

de Craen AJM. 'The human brain'. *Journal of Neurology, Neurosurgery and Psychiatry*. 2001; 71: 29–32.

Fiatarone-Singh MA. 'The effects of multi-dimensional home-based exercise on functional performance in the elderly'. *Journal of Gerontology*. 2003; 57A: M262–82.

Garg A. 'High-monounsaturated-fat diets for patients with diabetes mellitus: a meta-analysis'. *American Journal of Clinical Nutrition*. 1988; 67(3 suppl): 577S–582S.

Hass CJL, Garzarella D, De Hoyos D, Pollock ML. 'Single versus multiple sets in long-term recreational weightlifters'. *Medical Science Sports Exercise.* 2000; 32: 235–42.

Holmes MD, Chen WY, Feskanich D, et al. 'Physical activity and survival after breast cancer diagnosis'. *Journal of the American Medical Association.* 2005; 293: 2479–86.

Ireton-Jones CS and Snell PG. 'Weight training prevents the decrease in resting metabolic rate during moderate weight loss'. *Circulation.* 1990; 82: III–62.

Kasch FW, Boyer JL, Schmidt PK, et al. 'Ageing of the cardiovascular system during 33 years of aerobic exercise'. *Age & Ageing.* 1999; 28: 531–6.

Kritz-Silverstein D. 'Report on 11-year exercise study of 900 older athletes'. *American Journal of Epidemiology.* 2001; March 15: 596–603.

Levi F, Lucchini F, Negri E, et al. 'Trends in mortality from cardiovascular and cerebrovascular diseases in Europe and other areas of the world'. *Heart.* 2002; 88: 119–24.

Manson JE, Hu FB, Rich-Edwards JW, et al. 'A prospective study of walking as compared with vigorous exercise in the prevention of coronary heart disease in women'. *New England Journal of Medicine.* 1999; 341: 650–8.

McAuley KA, Williams SM, Mann JI, et al. 'Intensive lifestyle changes are necessary to improve insulin sensitivity: a randomised controlled trial'. *Diabetes Care.* 2002; 25(3): 445–52.

McGuire DK, Levine BD, Williamson JW, Snell PG, et al. 'A thirty-year follow-up of the Dallas Bedrest and Training Study: I. Effect of age on the cardiovascular response to exercise'. *Circulation.* 2001; 104: 1350–7.

Pollock ML, Foster C, Knapp D, et al. 'Effect of age and training on aerobic capacity and body composition of Master athletes'. *Journal of Applied Physiology.* 1987; 62: 725–31.

Pollock ML, Graves JE, Swart DL, Lowenthal DT. 'Exercise training and prescription for the elderly'. *Southern Medical Association Journal.* 1994; 87: S88–95.

Pollock ML, Mengelkoch LJ, Graves JE, Lowenthal DT, Limacher MC, Foster C, Wilmore JH. 'Twenty-year follow-up of aerobic power and body composition of older track athletes'. *Journal of Applied Physiology.* 1997; 82(5): 1508–16.

Rehm J, Room R, Graham K, Monteiro M, et al. 'The relationship of average volume of alcohol consumption and patterns of drinking to burden of disease: an overview'. *Addiction.* 2003; 98(9): 1209–28.

Ridker PM, Cushman M, Stampfer MJ, et al. 'Inflammation, aspirin, and the risk of cardiovascular disease in apparently healthy men'. *New England Journal of Medicine.* 2000; 336: 973–9.

Sohn RS and Micheli LJ. 'The effect of running on the pathogenesis of osteoarthritis of the hips and knees'. *Clinical Orthopaedics & Related Research*. 1985; 198: 106–9.

Thompson PD, Funk EJ, Carleton RA, Sturner WQ. 'Incidence of death during jogging in Rhode Island from 1975 through 1980'. *Journal of the American Medical Association*. 1982; 247(18): 2535–8.

Tuomilehto J, Lindstrom J, Eriksson JG, et al. 'Finnish Diabetes Prevention Study Group: prevention of type 2 diabetes mellitus by changes in lifestyle among subjects with impaired glucose tolerance'. *New England Journal of Medicine*. 2001; 344: 1343–50.

Vincent KR, Braith RW, Feldman RA, et al. 'Improved cardiorespiratory endurance following 6 months of resistance exercise in elderly men and women'. *Arch Intern Med*. 2002; 162: 673–8.

The following journals were also consulted for various articles: *Journal of Aging and Physical Activity*, *Brain Research*, *Australian and New Zealand Journal of Public Health*.

Quizzes

Third Age quiz

Disagree = 1, agree =2, strongly agree =3

1. I worry about not being able to do activities I enjoy as I grow older. _____
2. I am aware of declining physical and mental abilities. _____
3. The thought of growing old and dependent on others frightens me. _____
4. I devote more time and energy to improving my fitness and health. _____
5. Keeping active and physically independent is important to me.

Total score _____

Interpretation

5–8: You need a wake-up call. You are passive about your declining abilities and will fade away without a whimper.

9–11: You are doing okay but should do more.

12–15: You are highly motivated to get the most out of the Third Age. You have already put into practice the advice in this book.

Nutrition and activity quiz

Tick Yes or No next to each question and see how you can keep living smart.

NO YES

☐ ☐ I eat at least five servings of fruit and vegetables every day.

☐ ☐ I eat at least six servings of bread, rice, pasta and cereal every day.

☐ ☐ I drink or eat reduced-fat or fat-free milk and yoghurt, and seldom eat high-fat cheese.

☐ ☐ I rarely eat high-fat meat like bacon, hot dogs, sausage, or mince.

☐ ☐ I take it easy on high-fat baked goods such as pies, cakes, biscuits, pastries and doughnuts.

☐ ☐ I rarely add butter, margarine, oil, sour cream or mayonnaise to foods when I'm cooking or at the table.

☐ ☐ I rarely (less than twice a week) eat fried foods.

☐ ☐ I try to maintain a healthy weight.

☐ ☐ I am physically active for at least thirty minutes on most days of the week.

☐ ☐ I usually take the stairs instead of waiting for an elevator.

☐ ☐ I try to spend most of my free time being active, instead of watching television or sitting at the computer.

☐ ☐ I never or only occasionally drink alcohol.

Results

If you answered Yes to 4 or fewer questions you are on Diet Alert. Your diet is probably too high in fat and too low in plant foods like fruit, vegetables and grains. You need to look at your eating habits and find ways to make some changes.

If you answered Yes to between 5 and 8 questions, you're halfway there. Look at your No answers to decide where your diet needs changing.

If you answered Yes to 9 or more questions you are living smart. Don't change your diet.

Biological age quiz

Section A: Chronological age
1. What is your current age (in years)?

_____ Total Score (Section A)

Section B: Dietary choices

2. How frequently do you eat fried, grilled or barbecued foods?

Often	Once a day	Few times a week	Once a week	Almost never
4	3	2	1	-2

3. How often do you consume nutritional oils (not fried or heated)?

Never	Once a week	Once a day	2+ times a day
2	1	0	-1

4. How many servings of fruits or vegetables do you consume? (1 serving = 1 cup.)

Almost never	Few times a week	One a day	3 a day	5+ a day
3	2	1	-1	-2

5. How often do you consume whole grains and/or natural fibre? (Example: whole wheat, brown or wild rice.)

Almost never	Once a week	Few times a week	Often
3	2	1	-2

6. How many glasses of water do you consume daily? (Water does not include coffee, black tea, soft drinks or alcohol.)

Almost never	One a day	4 a day	8 a day	10+ a day
3	2	1	0	-2

7. Do you consume sugar, soda, white flour or other processed food? (Example: canned foods, fast food, TV dinners, foods with preservatives added.)

3+ times a day	Once a day	Few times a week	Almost never
3	2	1	-1

8. How many alcoholic drinks do you consume per week?

12+	8	4	2	Almost never
3	2	1	0	-1

9. How often do you add salt to your food?

All food	Daily	Few times a week	Once a month	Almost never
3	2	1	0	−1

_____ Total Score (Section B)

Section C: Dietary supplementation

10. Do you take a multivitamin?

Almost never	Once a week	Few times a week	Daily
2	1	0	−1

11. Do you take antioxidants? (Example: grape-seed extract, selenium.)

Almost never	Once a week	Few times a week	Daily
2	1	0	−1

_____ Total Score (Section C)

Section D: Daily activities

12. Do you exercise? (Thirty or more minutes of continuous activity or increments of at least 10 minutes.)

Almost never	Once a week	3 times a week	5+ times a week
3	2	−2	−3

13. When you exercise, do you do so for more than two hours? (If you do not exercise, please put '0' as your answer.)

Most times	50% of the time	Almost never
4	2	0

14. Do you sleep well and awake rested?

Almost never	Sometimes	Usually	Always
3	2	0	−1

15. How often do you have normal bowel movements?

Once a week	Every 4 days	Every second day	Daily	2+ times a day
4	3	2	0	−2

_____ Total Score (Section D)

Section E: Medical history

16. Is there a history of the following conditions in your family? Cancer, diabetes, heart disease, depression, obesity, liver disease, high cholesterol, high blood pressure.

2 or more	One	None
1	0	−1

17. Have you ever had any of the following conditions? Cancer, diabetes, heart disease, depression, obesity, liver disease, high cholesterol, high blood pressure.

2 or more	One	None
3	2	−2

18. How frequently do you experience the following conditions? Headache, fever, sore throat, muscle aches (not exercise induced) colds or flu, rash, swelling.

Once a day	Once a week	Once a month	Almost never
3	2	0	−1

19. Have you ever been exposed to heavy metals or toxic substances? (Example: mechanics, hair dresser, nail technician, etc.)

Daily	Weekly	Monthly	Almost never
4	3	2	0

20. Have you been exposed to heavy metals via dentalwork of fillings?

3+ fillings	2 fillings	1 filling	Never
4	3	2	0

_____ Total Score (Section E)

Section F: Stress

21. How many full meals do you eat a day? (A snack is not a full meal.)

Never	4+ a day	3 a day	2 a day	One a day
3	3	0	−1	−2

22. At work or at home, how often are you in front of electronic equipment? (Example: computers, television, live cameras, electrical wires.)

8+ hours a day	6+ hours a day	Few hours a day	Almost never
3	2	1	0

23. How often are you exposed to cigarette smoke (direct or second hand)?

All day	Few times a day	Few times a week	Almost never
4	3	1	−1

24. Do you use recreational or street drugs?

2+ times a day	Once a day	Once a week	Once a month	Never
4	3	2	1	0

25. Do you drive in heavy traffic?

For a living	Daily (3+ hours)	Daily (1–2 hours)	Almost never
3	2	1	−1

26. At work and/or home, do you experience stress?

Very high	High	Moderate	Slight	Almost none
4	3	2	1	−2

_____ Total Score (Section F)

Calculating your biological age

Add your scores from the following sections together to calculate you biological age.

Section A: Chronological Age   _____

Section B: Dietary Choices   _____

Section C: Dietary Supplementation   _____

Section D: Daily Activities   _____

Section E: Medical History   _____

Section F: Stress   _____

Total   _____